Behavioral Evaluation of Hearing in Infants and Young Children

Jane R. Madell, Ph.D.

Director, Communicative Disorders
Department of Otolaryngology
Long Island College Hospital
Brooklyn, New York
Professor, Clinical Otolaryngology
State University of New York
Health Sciences Center
Brooklyn, New York

1998
Thieme
New York · Stuttgart

Thieme New York
333 Seventh Avenue
New York, NY 10001

Behavioral Evaluation of Hearing in Infants and Young Children
Jane R. Madell, Ph.D.

Library of Congress Cataloging-in-Publication Data

Madell, Jane Reger.
   Behavioral evaluation of hearing in infants and young children /
Jane R. Madell.
       p.   cm.
   Includes bibliographical references and index.
   ISBN 0-86577-692-X (TNY). —ISBN 3-13-107981-9 (GTV)
   1. Hearing disorders in infants—Diagnosis. 2. Hearing disorders
in children—Diagnosis. 3. Behavioral assessment of infants.
4. Behavioral assessment of children. 5. Audiometry. I. Title.
   [DNLM: 1. Hearing Tests—in infancy & childhood. 2. Hearing
Tests—methods. 3. Hearing Disorders—in infancy & childhood.
4. Hearing Disorders—diagnosis. 5. Behavior—in infancy &
childhood.   WV 272 M181b 1998]
   RF291.5.C45M33   1998
   G18.92'0978—dc21
   DNLM/DLC
   for Library of Congress   98-4647
                                                                   CIP

Important note: Medical knowledge is ever-changing. As new research and clinical experience broaden our knowledge, changes in treatment and drug therapy may be required. The authors and the editors of the material herein have consulted sources believed to be reliable in their efforts to provide information that is complete and in accord with the standards accepted at the time of publication. However, in view of the possibility of human error by the authors, editors, or publisher of the work herein, or changes in medical knowledge, neither the authors, editors, publisher, nor any other party who has been involved in the preparation of this work, warrants that the information contained herein is in every respect accurate or complete, and they are not responsible for any errors or omissions or for the results obtained from use of such information. Readers are encouraged to confirm the information contained herein with other sources. For example, readers are advised to check the product information sheet included in the package of each drug they plan to administer to be certain that the information contained in this publication is accurate and that changes have not been made in the recommended dose or in the contraindications for administration. This recommendation is of particular importance in connection with new or infrequently used drugs.

Some of the product names, patents, and registered designs referred to in this book are in fact registered trademarks or proprietary names even though specific reference to this fact is not always made in the text. Therefore, the appearance of a name without designation as proprietary is not to be construed as a representation by the publisher that it is in the public domain.

Printed in the United States of America
Composition by Compset, Inc.; Printed by Hamilton Printing Company

5 4 3 2 1

TNY ISBN 0-86577-692-X
GTV ISBN 3-13-107981-9

For Rob, Jody, and Josh, who make every day worth living!

Contents

Appendices

Foreword

How gratifying it is to have someone restore behavioral testing of infants to respectability! And Dr. Jane Madell is the most appropriate person to do that. She has been a warrior in the battle to obtain the very best diagnosis and amplification for the child with hearing impairment. She fought for combining the best technology with knowledgeable behavioral testing and clinical observations; she fought for nonconventional hearing aids for children who required atypical fittings; and she fought to tailor-make the intervention program to the child's needs. What she has is that mystical rapport with children that marks a great clinician.

Audiology actually began as an art, like medicine—the art of personal rapport with clients or patients. Even in the early days of audiology in the army, it was a hands-on, one-on-one relationship with hearing impaired individuals. The diagnosis of a hearing loss, the hearing aid fitting, and the ultimate auditory rehabilitation, relied on a personal bond between the clinician and client. When younger and younger children were gathered into the audiologist's venue it became even more important to have that personal bond between the child and the clinician. That was perhaps why, initially, women were more at ease than men in generating the necessary rapport. Lady Irene Ewing of England was the forerunner of behavioral testing with children, developing in the 1940's the distraction test with noisemakers that was to become a staple in the public health system of England for six-month olds. To my mind, it was unfortunate that this procedure became so officially implanted that it became difficult in England to supplant it with screening at birth using electrophysiological techniques. In the U.S., the National Joint Committee on Newborn Hearing prevented such kinds of screening from becoming established, recommending as early as 1980 that electrophysiological techniques be employed for newborn screening. This action points out the difference between the use of behavioral tests by audiologists for diagnostic purposes, and their use as mass screening devices. The latter testing requires well-established sensitivity/specificity ratios before acceptance. Behavioral testing of infants by trained clinicians, on the other hand, is a requisite and well-recognized procedure.

Behavioral testing of infants progressed rapidly. As early as 1950 we find women like Doreen Pollack and a colleague using a manual VRA test with young children: one tester stood by a window and popped up a doll whenever the tone was responded to by the child!

At this time some men were reporting on variations of the VRA technique: Dix and Hallpike in England developed a "Peep Show" in 1947, with the child uncovering a picture when the tone was heard. In the U.S., C. Olaf Haug modified this procedure by developing an instrument, the "Pediacoumeter", where the child controls the appearance of a toy when he or she hears the tone.

When Mrs. Pollack joined the staff at the University of Denver in 1952, we experienced more and more with behavioral testing. We even tried the then-popular PGSR test that William Hardy had reported from Johns Hopkins Hospital. But after extensive use of this instrument (without employing shock conditions), we found that our observations of the infants' responses were more reliable than the PGSR! On infants under 18 months we used the type of behavioral observations that Dr. Madell has so well described and that every clinician should become comfortable with. Of course, children over that age could be conditioned to some sort of play conditioning audiometry.

I was greatly amused just a few years ago when a neurologist/ABR technician, reporting on ABR with infants, stated, "And now, with this new technique, babies under a year old can, for the first time, be fitted with hearing aids because of the accuracy to fit hearing aids of children under a year of age—frequently under six months. Had we sat around waiting for ABR to appear, many people in their thirties would not now be as competent as they are in speech and language skills.

Fitting a hearing aid on an infant has indeed been simplified by the use of ABR testing. But such testing still requires confirmation with behavioral observations, not only of the level of hearing, but of the responses of the child to the use of the aid. Anyone who would fit a hearing aid to an infant on the basis of ABR responses alone cannot be considered a clinician.

The miracles of technology have given us welcome testing procedures to add to our armamentarium: ABR, OAE, Immittance meters; these add credibility to our profession. However, Dr. Jerry Northern has questioned just how long they will be in our exclusive proprietorship: there is already a home testing instrument (the "EarCheck Monitor") that replaces the Immittance meter; an infant screening system (the "Clarity"), that measures both automated ABR and otoacoustic emissions, operable by non-audiologists. There is even a "Personal Hearing Screener" designed to permit the general public to screen their own hearing. And the MRI has replaced the ABR as the gold standard measurement of acoustic nerve tumors. Northern states that we must strengthen our "people skills", confirming our competence as rehabilitationists and proving that our audiologic "treatments" *do* improve patient outcomes.

This book should help to restore the *art* of pediatric audiology—that undefinable empathy and understanding of the child that goes with true caring. It can be developed: read this book, and then test 100 normal-hearing children using the techniques Dr. Madell describes. Remembering that a hearing-impaired child is a normal child with normal responses once his threshold is reached, you will become comfortable with this remarkable *Art of Audiology*!

Marion P. Downs, Dr.H.S.
Professor Emerita
Department of Otolaryngology
University of Colorado
School of Medicine
Denver, Colorado

Acknowledgments

No one person ever writes a book alone. Even if one person puts the words on paper many people are involved in the process. I can say with certainty that this book could not have been written without the help and influences of many people. I have been fortunate to have many academic and clinical mentors during the course of my career. As an undergraduate student, David Luterman and Audrey Holland taught me to believe that there was no such thing as an untestable child. Claude Hayes and Charles Tait confirmed this for me when I got to graduate school. I learned from them that I would have to say "I cannot test this child" rather than "this child is untestable." Once we assigned the responsibility to the right person the task became more clear. Robert Goldstein taught me the value of precise and careful planning in both research and clinical work (and scheduled meetings at 6 AM to discuss it). In recent years, Mark Ross has continued to make me think and grow professionally.

In 30 years you get to work with a lot of people. If you are lucky, you learn from them. I was very lucky. I learned a great deal from the numerous audiologists, speech-language pathologists, psychologists, otolaryngologists, engineers, technicians and students with whom I had the good fortune to work. Perhaps the people from whom I have learned the most are the hearing impaired and difficult-to-test infants and children, and their families who helped me to learn, pushed me to find answers, refused to accept "I don't know," and, as a result, taught me to become a better clinician. This book belongs to them as much as to me.

None of the work I have done would have been possible without the support and love of my very special family. My husband, Rob, and my children Jody and Josh, supported and encouraged me and allowed me to develop into the clinician I wanted to be by not questioning my long hours and need to be away from home even before it was considered acceptable to be both a "professional" and a "mom."

Finally, I want to thank my secretary, Ruth Pacheco, who checked my spelling and made the pages look good, my friends and colleagues Laura Wilbur and Tziona Bin-Nun, who read the chapters and made valuable suggestions, and my editor, Andrea Seils, who put up with a variety of delays and offered many helpful suggestions to bring about the final product.

Jane R. Madell

1

The Role of Behavioral Testing in the Evaluation of Hearing in Infants

There is general agreement that hearing loss and other disabilities should be identified as early as possible to permit early remediation. Hearing is the primary avenue for language learning, social communication and interaction, and education (Fry, 1978; Hayes & Northern, 1996; Ross, Bracket, & Maxon, 1982) and the reduced ability to hear has a negative effect on all of these. Prelingual hearing loss is, in fact, two disabilities: hearing loss and language delay (Mauk, White, Mortensen, & Behrens, 1991; Allen & Schubert-Sudia, 1990; Yoshinaga-Itano, 1987). There is little disagreement that, regardless of the educational system in which parents choose to educate their hearing-impaired infants, all infants with hearing loss are best served when their hearing losses are identified early, and they are fitted with appropriate amplification and provided appropriate habilitation.

Early Language Learning

Early identification is critical because many speech perception activities begin very early. By 8 weeks of age, infants can distinguish the language spoken in their environment from other languages (Leonard, 1991); by 18 weeks, they can associate auditory information with visual information (e.g., recognize the oral posture associated with a vowel [Kuhl & Meltzoff, 1988]). Infants learn basic sounds of language by 6 months (Kuhl & Meltzoff, 1988), and by 7 months can detect major syntactic boundaries (recognize pauses). Children do not say first words until the second year of life, but by the end of the first year they know a great deal about language, so even before they say their first word, children are actively sorting out the sounds in the language to which they are exposed. Language is the single best predictor of future cognition in children and each month that passes in the first year without hearing could well represent a loss of language learning and of an opportunity to provide compensatory skills. (Rosetti, 1991).

Evaluation of identification patterns of hearing-impaired infants indicates that hearing loss is frequently not identified until the second year. The Joint Committee on Infant Hearing (1994) recommended that hearing be screened by 3 months, or at the latest, by 6 months, and that the diagnostic process be completed and rehabilitation begun by age 6 months. The National Institutes of Health has recommended newborn hearing screening before hospital discharge; however, the literature has a significant number of reports verifying the delay in identification (Coplan, 1987; Elssman, Matkin, & Sabo, 1987; Luterman & Chasin, 1970; Madell & Hoffman, 1987; Parving, 1984). Stein, Clark, & Kraus, 1983; Stein, Jabaley, Spitz, Stoakley, & McGee, 1990 reported that the mean age of enrollment in habilitation programs was 20 months for neonatal intensive care unit (NICU) graduates and 19.6 months for graduates of the well baby nursery. The Utah high-risk hearing screening program (Mahoney & Eichwald, 1986) reported identification of hearing-impaired infants was made by 7.6 months and amplification fitted by 9.8 months. However, in Arizona and other states, identification of hearing loss is at close to 19 months and amplification fitting at 25 months (Elssmann et al, 1987), similar to the results reported by Stein et al (1990).

The Effect of Hearing Loss

The effect of hearing loss should not be underestimated. Almost any hearing loss has a negative impact on language learning and academic development. Obviously, the more severe the hearing loss is, the more serious will be the impact. However, even children with mild conductive or unilateral hearing losses have demonstrated communicative and academic problems (Northern & Downs, 1984; Bess, Klee, & 1986; Davis, Elfeinbein, Schum, & Bentler, 1986; Davis, 1990; Rosenfeld & Madell, 1996).

Early Identification

Recent advances in hearing screening (otoacoustic emissions and auditory brainstem response testing) have increased interest in hearing in infants and have encouraged audiologists, pediatricians, and parents to identify hearing loss early. The new hearing screening techniques can identify that a problem may be present, but they do not provide sufficient information to identify accurately the degree of hearing loss across frequencies, and to fit amplification, both of which are essential before initiating a habilitation program. To fit amplification accurately and appropriately, it is essential to have a frequency-specific and ear-specific audiogram, and at this time, these audiograms cannot be provided using electrophysiological techniques. Behavioral testing, in fact, continues to be the so-called gold standard for determining hearing thresholds.

In spite of the available technology, identification of hearing loss in infants continues to be delayed beyond the ideal time of 6 months of age recommended by the Joint Committee on Infant Hearing (1994). The high-risk register can only identify 50% of infants with hearing loss (Mauk et al, 1991). Infant hearing screening, although not yet universal, offers the opportunity to identify infants at risk, however, even when such infants are identified, the obvious next step, fitting amplification, is frequently delayed, partly because many audiologists do not feel comfortable assessing hearing in infants. Improved confidence by audiologists of their ability to identify hearing loss accurately in infants is needed. In the 30 years during which I have been evaluating hearing in infants and young children, I have come to believe firmly that every infant can be tested for hearing loss within a reasonably short period of time. Not every audiologist feels comfortable working with infants. Even those who do it on a regular basis may not feel completely confident working with newborns, sick infants, or children who are difficult to test. With experience, however, audiologists can become comfortable working with infants and develop reliable testing skills. The flexibility of current amplification systems allows audiologists to change the amplification signal as more information about the child's auditory status becomes available.

The Pediatric Working Group (1996) has suggested that behavioral testing is not the preferred method of hearing evaluation when the purpose is to select hearing aids for children younger than 6 months because of (a) prolonged cooperation required from the child, (b) excessive test time needed, (c) poor frequency resolution, and (d) poor test–retest reliability. There is no doubt that the evaluation of hearing in infants and young children is time consuming and can require prolonged cooperation, but we should not exclude behavioral testing for these reasons. If we believe that the information obtained from behavioral testing is valuable, if not critical, our goal should be, rather, to develop procedures that will provide reliable behavioral test results. We would not make a determination about auditory function or fit amplification on a normally developing five-year-old without first obtaining a good behavioral audiogram, and for good reason: The behavioral audiogram gives us valuable information. Within certain limits, it should be possible to obtain good behavioral evaluations on children of any age or developmental status.

It is my hope that the information in this book and its accompanying video will assist audiologists in developing the skills necessary to feel comfortable in assessing hearing in infants and children who are difficult to test.

References and Readings

Allen, M.C., & Schubert-Sudia, S.E. (1990). Prevention of prelingual hearing impairment. *Semin Hear, 11*, 134–148.

American Speech-Language-Hearing Association. (1994). Joint Committee on Infant Hearing, 1994 position statement. *ASHA, 36*, 38–41.

Bess, F.M., & Klee, T.M. (1986). Unilateral sensorineural hearing loss in children. *Ear Hear, 7*, 3–54.

Coplan, J. (1987). Deafness: Ever heard of it? Delayed recognition of permanent hearing loss. *Pediatrics, 79*, 206–213.

Davis, J., Elfeinbein, J., Schum, R., & Bentler, R. (1986). Effects of mild and moderate hearing impairments on language, educational and psychosocial behavior of children. *J Speech Hear Disord, 51*, 53–62.

Davis, J. (1990). *Our Forgotten Children: Hard of Hearing Pupils in the Schools*, Bethesda, MD: Self Help for Hearing People.

Elssmann, S.F., Matkin, N.D., & Sabo, M.P. (1987). Early identification of congenital sensorineural hearing impairment. *J Hear, 40*, 13–17.

Flexor, C. (1996). *Amplification for Young Children: Case Studies*. Salt Lake City, UT: American Academy of Audiology.

Fry, D. (1978). The role and primacy of the auditory channel in speech and language development. In Ross, M., & Giolas, T. (eds.): *Auditory Management of Hearing Impaired Children*. Baltimore: University Park Press.

Hayes, D., & Northern, J. (1996). *Infants and Hearing*. San Diego, CA: Singular Publishing.

Kuhl, P., & Meltzoff, A. (1988). Speech as an intermodal object of perception. In Yonas, A. (ed.): *Perceptual Development in Infancy* (pp. 235–266). Hillsdale, NJ: Lawrence Erlbaum.

Leonard, L.B. (1991). New trends in the study of early language acquisition. *ASHA, 4*, 43–44.

Luterman, D., & Chasin, J. (1970). The pediatrician and the parent of the deaf child. *Pediatrics, 79*, 115–116.

Madell, J.R., & Hoffman, R.A. (1987). Delay in pediatric referral for audiologic evaluation. Paper presented at the American-Speech-Language-Hearing Association (ASHA) Convention, Chicago, IL, November, 1987.

Mauk, G.A., White, K.R., Mortensen, L.B., & Behrens, T.R. (1991). The effectiveness of screening programs based on high-risk characteristics in early identification of hearing impairment. *Ear and Hear, 12*, 312–318.

Mahoney, T.M., & Eichwald, J.G. (1987). The ups and "Downs" of high-risk screening: The Utah statewide program. *Semin Hear, 8*, 155–163.

Northern, J. & Downs, M. (1984). *Hearing in Children* (3rd ed.). Baltimore: Williams & Wilkins.

Parving, A. (1984). Early detection and identification of congenital/early acquired hearing disability. Who takes the initiative? *Int J Pediatr Otorhinolaryngol, 2*, 107–117.

The Pediatric Working Group of the Conference on Amplification for Children with Auditory Deficits (1996). Amplification for infants and children with hearing loss. *Am J Audiol, 5*, 53–68.

Rosenfeld, R.M., & Madell, J.R. (1996). Auditory function in normal hearing children with middle ear effusion. In Lim, D., Bluestone, C., Casselbrant, M., Klein, J., & Ogra, P. (eds.): *Recent Advances in Otitis Media*. Hamilton, Ontario: Decker.

Ross, M., Brackett, D., & Maxon, A. (1982). *Hard of Hearing Children in Regular Schools*. Englewood Cliffs, NJ: Prentice-Hall.

Rossetti, L. (1991). Communication assessment: Birth to 36 months. *ASHA, 33*, 45–44.

Stein, L., Clark, S., & Kraus, N. (1983). The hearing-impaired infant: Patterns of identification and habilitation. *Ear Hear, 4*, 232–236.

Stein, L., Jabaley, T., Spitz, R., Stoakley, D., & McGee, T. (1990). The hearing-impaired infant: Patterns of identification and habilitation revisited. *Ear Hear, 11*, 201–205.

Yoshinaga-Itano, C. (1987). Aural habilitation: A key to acquisition of knowledge, language, and speech. *Semin Hear, 8*, 169–174.

2

Obtaining a Case History

A good case history is a valuable tool and an often-overlooked part of an audiological evaluation. All diagnosticians recognize the need to obtain some information before beginning testing, but the information obtained may not be sufficient, and the amount needed will vary according to the reason for the evaluation. If a child is scheduled for insertion of pressure equalization tubes and the evaluation is pre- or postsurgical, it may not be necessary to obtain an extensive history. However, if the child is being evaluated because of concern about hearing, speech or language development; developmental delay; or problems in school, then an extensive history is needed. Failure to obtain a sufficient history may reduce the information obtained from the evaluation and reduce the role of the evaluation and the evaluator to a technical one rather then a professional and diagnostic one.

Taking a history obviously provides information necessary to learn about a child's development and health, but it also provides an opportunity to observe the child and to get to know the family and the caregivers and to understand their concerns and needs, and to assess their objectivity. If different family members have different viewpoints, this frequently comes out during the interview process. The time spent obtaining a history also provides an opportunity to observe the child's interactions with family members and others and may uncover differences of opinion between your observations and those of the family members. Taking a history provides an excellent opportunity to develop rapport with and insights into the family, which may increase their willingness to accept your assessment results and recommendations for management.

By the end of the interview, the audiologist should have a good picture of the child's cognitive and developmental status and an initial estimate of the child's auditory skills. This information is critical for selecting appropriate test protocols; Without it, the audiologist may fail to recognize that although the child may be 4 years old chronologically, she or he is about 2 years old cognitively, which changes the appropriate test protocol from play to visual reinforcement audiometry. Using the wrong test protocol is not only inefficient, but can cause errors in determining auditory status. For example, attempting to use play for a child who is not cognitively ready for the task may make it appear that the child is not hearing when, in fact, the problem is that the child cannot perform the task.

Collecting History Information

Some clinics mail out questionnaires in advance and have families complete them before coming in for evaluation. This method allows the family to think about answers, to check with other family members or clinicians if needed, and to find the addresses of healthcare providers and schools for example. This is especially helpful if someone other than the parents (e.g., babysitter, grandparents, foster parents) brings the child to the evaluation. If the child is a foster child, mailing out the questionnaire in advance allows the social service agency responsible to provide the necessary information. However, not all families will complete forms even if they are received in advance.

Some programs give families questionnaires to complete when they arrive at the center before being seen for evaluation. Although this method limits the time for completing the form and for thinking about the answers, and does not permit obtaining information that is not easily recalled, it ensures that some information will be obtained. However, even when history information forms are completed by the family, the clinical still needs to ask questions and to spend time reviewing the information before initiating testing. This review frequently uncovers blank spaces or incomplete answers that need to be completed before testing can begin. Some clinicians prefer to collect history information by asking all the questions themselves. Although this method allows the clinician to direct the questions, as needed, and to expand or to delete questions in certain areas, it extends the time needed for an evaluation because all information needs to be obtained at the time of the interview.

There are basic areas that should be reviewed in any history. Other questions will present themselves as the interviewer learns more about the child and the concerns of the parents or caregivers. A printed history form is frequently useful because it provides basic information (see Appendices 2, 3, and 4), but it is important not to let the form limit the questions. The form should simply be viewed simply as a guide.

Topics To Be Covered

A complete history covers several different areas and, depending on the reason for the evaluation, emphasizes different parts of the history. For example, if this evaluation is an initial one or if the child has not been seen recently, the obvious first question is, "Why have you brought your child here today?" By determining the reason for the visit the evaluator can find out what the parent or caregiver's concerns are and begin to get a picture of the goals of the evaluation. The next step is obtaining specific information.

Pregnancy and Birth History

It is usually easiest to begin by obtaining pregnancy and birth history, finding out if there were any complications or illnesses during the pregnancy or delivery that might have had an impact on hearing or development (see Appendices 2 and 3). Information about previous pregnancies can also be important. Previous pregnancies that resulted in miscarriages or produced children with developmental disabilities, may suggest the need for genetic counseling. Obtaining information about the length of hospitalization for the birth may provide insight into difficulties that were present and offers an opportunity to inquire about medications and drugs (prescription, over-the-counter, and illegal) taken during or immediately before the pregnancy that may have affected the fetus.

Health History

The health history determines if there is reason for concern about acquired or progressive hearing loss or other developmental conditions. Information should be obtained about ear infections and allergies, which might have an impact on conductive hearing loss, and about high fever, meningitis, other viruses, and medication or vaccine reactions, which might have an impact on sensorineural hearing loss. For example, the evaluator might ask if the parents were aware of any change in hearing, motor skills, or development after an illness or vaccination. Other health issues, such as feeding problems, seizures, and so forth, should also be explored at this time.

Developmental History

It is critical to explore the child's developmental history so that the audiologist knows the child's developmental age and can select the appropriate test protocol and obtain accurate test results. A carefully obtained developmental history also provides information useful in sorting out different communication disorders (e.g., hearing loss, developmental delay, pervasive developmental disability). The ability to recognize the presence of one of these conditions also permits the selection of test techniques that facilitate obtaining accurate hearing test results.

Obtaining specific information about motor development is critical. If the child's motor milestones are on target, some developmental and neurological disorders can be ruled out, but if they are delayed, the child may have a developmental or a neurological disorder that is contributing to a speech and language delay. If the child is walking, but is clumsy and falls a lot, a neurological evaluation may be indicated. It may also be useful to ask whether the child's hearing changes after a fall, which may suggest the need for a neuro-otologic evaluation for perilymph fistula.

Information about eating, feeding, and swallowing should be obtained in this section and will provide a more complete picture of the child. Age at toilet training is also useful information. For example, if a child is 4 years old and not yet toilet trained, this area may require some further evaluation.

To get a good picture of the child's developmental level it is sometimes helpful to ask the parents to make a judgment. A useful question is, "If you were a relative visiting from out of town and did not know the child's age, how old would you think she or he is from observing how she or he behaves?" This provides a lot of information and can add to what you know about the child, provide information about the parents perspective, uncover differences in points of view of different family members, and assist in counseling.

Communication History: Hearing

It is frequently useful to begin by asking what the parents think about the child's hearing. They may answer that the child's hearing is fine, or that he or she "hears when he or she wants to." The clinician can assist the parents in developing a better picture of the child's hearing by asking specific questions. Does the child respond to sounds that are out of sight (doorbell, television [TV], or water running in the bathtub from another room, a key in the door, being called from another room)? Can she or he distinguish between the doorbell and the phone? Does he or she want the TV or radio turned loud? Does it matter if the TV sound is on or off? Does he or she respond to sound change, or does he or she hear better at some times than at others? When does this happen? Is the change associated with a cold or a fall? Are some sounds uncomfortable for the child? Is he or she afraid of some sounds and if so, which ones and under what circumstances? If the child is afraid of someone yelling or of a baby crying, it may be a reasonable reaction to the situation and not an indication of a hearing problem.

Does the child wear hearing aids, an FM system, or both? If so, which ones, at what settings, when were they obtained, and most important, how does the child function with them? Is the family satisfied with the amplification? How often is the child's hearing tested and how often has the child's amplification been changed? If it has been changed frequently it may indicate changes in hearing or difficulty in accepting auditory abilities.

Communication History: Speech and Language

The communication history provides information about the child's speech and language development. Did the child babble? When? What kinds of sounds did the child make? Did the babbling change, or stop? When did the child say his or her first word? What was it and was it really a word? For example, if the babbling was "mamama" some parents think that the child is saying "mama" when in fact she or he is just babbling. It is necessary to ask how the parents knew that the child was referring to or calling mother when she or he said "mamama." When did the child begin to use phrases and sentences? Does the child understand verbal requests without use of gesture or situational cues? For example, if you hand the child a dirty diaper and say, "Throw it away," it is not clear whether the child is understanding the command from the situation or from the verbal directions. Does the child understand when there are no clues or when he or she cannot see the person's face? How does the child communicate needs? By speech? Gestures? Signs? By leading the person to what she or he wants? Did the child begin to speak and then stop speaking? If the child stopped speaking, it may indicate a progressive hearing loss or a developmental disorder such as autism or pervasive developmental disorder.

Social History

When did the child show an interest in others? Does he or she seek out other children and adults or prefer to play alone? What are the child's preferred play activities? Are they typical of a child of this age? How does the child get along with others? How does the child respond to others? Does she or he make eye contact? Have there been changes in the child's behavior? Was the child more responsive at an earlier age? A hearing-impaired child will be responsive to others, seek to play with children and adults, and play with toys appropriately if they are within his or her cognitive level. (Board games that require language for directions may pose a problem, but physical games should not.) A child with a developmental delay may do all the above but at a later age than normally developing children. A child with a pervasive developmental disability may not make eye contact, may not play with others, or may play with a restricted range of toys and play with them in a restricted fashion (such as playing with cars by spinning the wheels).

Educational History

It is useful to obtain information about where the child is currently in school, whether it is in a regular or special education program, what kinds of special services the child is receiving in school, and whether the family is satisfied with the school placement. It is also useful to inquire about previous schools and the reasons for a change. Some parents are unable to verbalize that their child has been diagnosed with a specific educational or learning problem but will provide information about schooling, which can be of assistance in learning more about the child.

Special Services

Information about what kinds of special services are available in school and outside of school is useful and provides insight into how the school and the family view the child. Services offered may include speech–language therapy, hearing (auditory training) therapy, occupational and physical therapy, psychological or psychiatric counseling, or educational tutoring.

Other Evaluations

Knowledge about other evaluations the child has had and their results provides important information about the child and may include previous audiological evaluations, amplification evaluations, speech and language evaluations, occupational and physical therapy evaluations, and psycho-educational evaluations. Information from medical evaluations, including otolaryngological, neurological, and psychiatric evaluations, is also useful. Review of information provided by other professionals adds to the picture and helps in understanding the child.

High-risk Register

It is important to know whether the child meets any of the criteria for hearing loss listed on the High-Risk Register (see Appendix 1). Most of the information should have been included in questions asked during the taking of a history, but if there are any doubts about whether the child meets any of the high-risk criteria, they should be resolved before completion of the evaluation.

Conclusion

Obtaining a history takes time but provides valuable information. At the very least, by the end of obtaining a history the audiologist should have a very good sense of the child's cognitive status and motor abilities, which are critical for selecting the appropriate test protocol (observation, visual reinforcement, or play audiometry), and of the child's speech and language and developmental levels, which are also useful in selecting test methods. During the evaluation, the audiologist determines if his or her initial impression was accurate or not. Information obtained from the history and from observation of the child should also give the audiologist a good idea of what to expect from the hearing evaluation. It may be helpful to try to estimate the audiogram from history information and from observation of the child before beginning the test. Doing so over a period of time will improve the audiologist's ability to take a history as well as the ability to make accurate observations of children.

References and Readings

Ehrlich, C. (1983). A case history for children. In Katz, J. (ed.): *Handbook of Clinical Audiology* (3rd ed., pp. 607–620). Baltimore: Williams & Wilkins.

Hayes, D., & Northern, J.L. (1996). *Infants and Hearing.* San Diego: Singular Publishing.

Matkin, N. (1984). Early recognition and referral of hearing impaired children. *Pediatr Rev, 6,* 153.

3

Preparing for the Evaluation

Selecting the Appropriate Test Protocol

A critical factor in obtaining reliable test results is selection of the appropriate test protocol. To do so, it is essential to know the child's cognitive level and the child's physical abilities. Knowledge of what the child is capable of before initiating testing is critical.

Cognitive Age

There are three behavioral techniques, each of which is appropriate for children at different levels: Observation audiometry is the appropriate technique for infants from birth to 6 months' cognitive age, visual reinforcement audiometry (VRA) is appropriate for infants from 6 months to 36 months, and play audiometry is appropriate for children 36 months and older, allowing for some flexibility at upper and lower age limits. Knowing the child's cognitive age allows the clinician to select the appropriate test method, which is essential. For example, it would not be a good idea, to ask a 2-month-old to raise his or her hand when he or she heard a sound. Doing so would lead to the conclusion that every 2-month-old child is deaf.

Unfortunately, it is not always possible to rely solely on chronological age to determine cognitive level. Although many children function at the same levels cognitively and chronologically, not all do. Much of the information obtained from the history will help determine cognitive level. If speech and language skills are at or close to age level, one can assume that chronological and cognitive ages are the same or relatively close. Unfortunately, because many children undergo hearing evaluations because they are not developing speech and language skills, other information is needed to determine cognitive level. Motor development can be a useful marker. If

Table 3–1.   Before Beginning to Test

1. Determine the child's cognitive age from:
   History
   Reports from other evaluations
   Infant screening scales
2. Evaluate the child's physical status in terms of:
   Upper-torso control
   Head and neck control
   Vision
   Ability to manipulate toys
3. Choose the test room setup:
   1 room with 1 audiologist
   2 rooms with 2 audiologists, or 1 audiologist and 1 test assistant
   2 rooms with 1 audiologist and 1 parent as assistant

a child's motor skills are at age level, the child is usually cognitively at or close to chronological level, at least for the purpose of tasks for testing hearing. If information is not available from other sources, a number of tests are available to assess developmental level (see Table 3–2).

It is not a good idea to use the trial-and-error method to choose a test protocol; this method may work some, but not all, of the time. If a child's cognitive and chronological levels are too far apart, using an inappropriate test may give the appearance of hearing loss when none exists, or yield inaccurate thresholds because the child will not respond appropriately to the test stimulus. If a child were chronologically at the age for play but was tested with VRA, he or she might respond to the VRA toy a few times but would likely become bored after a few presentations. The child might respond to the toy when loud sounds were presented, but would be unlikely to respond to soft sounds, giving the mistaken impression of not having heard them. It would be most unusual for a normally developing 3- or 4-year-old child to respond to VRA but not respond to play. Should this hap-

Table 3–2.   Tests for Assessing Developmental Level

Brigance, 1991	Brigance Developmental Scale
Furuno et al., 1984	Hawaii Early Learning Profile
Katoff et al., 1978	Kent Infant Development Scale
Blaire, 1975	Language Evaluation Scale
Pollack, 1997	Pollack Developmental Milestones Scale
Frankenburg & Dodds, 1967	The Denver Developmental Screening Test (DDST)

pen, the possibility that the child has a developmental disability should be considered. Choosing the wrong test protocol may not be just a temporary setback. When testing young children, time is a critical factor, and selecting the wrong protocol may mean lack of cooperation from the child for the additional time needed for testing.

Physical Status

Once a child's cognitive level has been established, the child's physical condition needs to be evaluated to be certain that the child is capable of performing the test tasks. For observation audiometry, we are primarily looking for changes in sucking, which is relatively easy to discern. Does the child suck? If yes, the evaluator can do the task. An infant may have an eating problem and receive food through feeding tubes but use a pacifier and thus sucking can be observed with the pacifier. However, if the infant does not suck, it is probably not possible to obtain reliable observation audiometry responses.

RA uses a conditioned head turn in response to presentation of a sound stimulus, which requires the child to have vision good enough to see the reinforcing toy and neck control sufficient to turn and to look for the reinforcing toy. This task is most often performed with the child sitting either in a highchair or on someone's lap. If the child cannot sit, she or he can be placed in a supported position, such as in an infant seat, so that she or he can still make a conditioned head turn. If the child cannot make a head turn, it is not possible to use VRA. If the child is too visually impaired to see the toy at the standard testing distance, it may be possible to move the child closer to the reinforcer (keeping calibration concerns in mind if testing is performed in soundfield), or to move the reinforcer closer to the child. If the child is blind or for some other reason cannot see the reinforcer, it is not possible to use standard VRA protocols. A creative audiologist may be able to come up with adaptive protocols. (See Chapter 7, Evaluation of Special Populations.)

Play audiometry requires that the child perform a motor task in response to the presentation of a sound. The ability to do this task is limited only by the creativity of the tester. If the child cannot hold a toy and drop it in a bucket, he or she may be able to blink, move a finger, or push a button, for example.

Specific test information about the various behavior protocols is discussed in the following chapters.

Setting Up the Test Room

Using a Two-Room Setup

There are a number of different ways to set up a test room for the evaluation of hearing in infants and young children. The most common is a two-room setup with an audiologist and an audiometer in one room, and the child, parents, and test assistant in the other (Fig. 3–1). When using this setup, it is essential that both the audiologist and the test assistant have a full view of the child. The audiologist, who is presenting the test stimuli, needs to be able to observe the child to know when to present stimuli and when not to (e.g., not when the child is fidgeting or trying to get out of the chair) and both testers must be able to judge the presence or absence of a response.

It is also important that the two testers be able to communicate. If possible, the test assistant should have an earphone to hear directions or suggestions from the audiologist in the test room. It is important that the test assistant know when the stimulus is being presented so that he or she knows whether to reinforce the child's response. For example, if a child looks toward the VRA toy when a sound has been presented, the test assistant should become enthusiastic, clapping and laughing. If the child looks toward the toy when there has been no test stimulus, the test assistant does not reinforce the response. If the test assistant does not have an earphone, the tester and test assistant must develop visual cues to ensure that they are communicating.

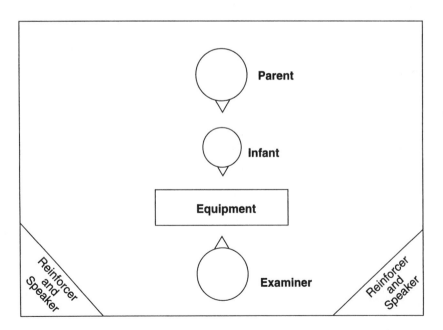

Figure 3–1. Two-room set-up.

Using a One-Room Test Setup

Some audiologists use a one-room test setup, either for all testing or for selected testing (Fig. 3–2). The advantage of a one-room test setup is that testing can be accomplished with only the audiologist, who now performs both the tester and test assistant roles and has more control. To accomplish this type of testing, the audiologist places the audiometer in the test room where the child will be. The setup should be arranged so that the child cannot see the audiometer controls and does not know when the interrupter switch is being pressed. The controls for the reinforcer toy for VRA also need to be located in a place not visible to the child. The audiologist can sit

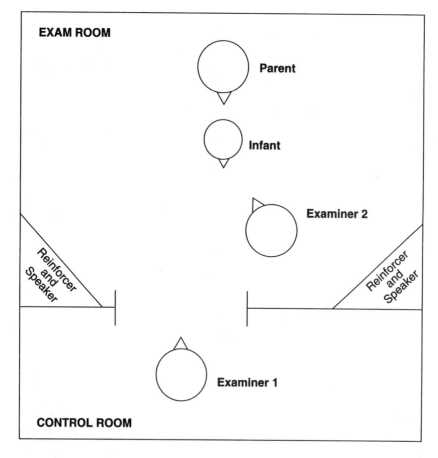

Figure 3–2. One-room set-up.

in front of the child and provide the stimulus, test assistance, as needed (such as handing the child toys for play audiometry or distracting the child for VRA), and reinforcement, as needed (either social or VRA). Even in centers where a two-room test setup is the norm, there are times when it is convenient to have the tester and child in the same room. For example, when testing children using play audiometry with earphones, it is often not necessary to have two testers: One tester and an audiometer can easily accomplish the task. Placing the audiometer out of the child's line of vision and is easily accomplished by seating the child at a test table with the audiologist seated next to the child, and the audiometer on a table or rolling cart behind the child, out of sight.

Experimenting with a variety of test setups will assist the audiologist in finding the one that is most comfortable for each test situation.

References and Readings

Blaire, F. (1975). *Language Evaluation Scale.* Milwaukee, WI: Department of Special Education, University of Wisconsin.

Brigance, A. (1991). *Diagnostic Inventory of Early Development.* North Billerica, MA: Curriculum Associates Incorporated.

Frankenburg, W., & Dodds, J. (1967). The Denver Developmental Screening Test. *J Pediatr, 71,* 181.

Furuno, S., O'Reilly, K.A., Hosaka, C.M., Inastuka, T.T., Zeisloft-Falbegy, B., & Allman, T. (1984). *Hawaii Early Learning Profile (Help Check List).* Palo Alst, CA: Vort Corporation.

Katoff, L., Reuter, J., & Dunn, V. (1978). *The Kent Infant Developmental Scale Manual.* Kent, OH: Kent State University.

Pollack, J. (1997). *Developmental Milestones Scale.* Brooklyn, NY: Lamm Institute, Long Island College Hospital.

4

Observation Audiometry: Testing Infants from Birth to 6 Months

The first, known use of neonatal hearing testing was in England in 1944, when Sir Alexander and Lady Irene Ewing used percussion sounds, teacups, and pitch pipes to elicit "aural reflex responses," reflex thresholds that were observable during the first 6 months but more difficult to observe as the infant grew older. Wedenberg began true infant screening in Sweden in 1956, using pure tones to elicit the auro-palpebral reflex. Froding continued Wedenberg's work, testing 2000 infants with sounds produced by a small gong and mallet, but was concerned about the lack of reliability of the response. The first large-scale program in the United States was a citywide hearing screening project in Denver conducted in 1964 by Marion Downs and Graham Sterrit with a hand-held noise generator that produced a 90-dB SPL noise centered at 3000 Hz. Although these methods identified some hearing impaired children, many were missed.

In an effort to improve infant hearing testing, Marion Downs requested that the American Speech-Language-Hearing Association (ASHA) organize the Joint Committee on Infant Hearing composed of members of ASHA, of the American Academy of Pediatrics, and of the American Academy of Ophthalmology and Otolaryngology. The Committee reviewed infant-hearing test protocols and developed a high-risk register. For many years, only infants identified through the high-risk register were screened, but in time, audiologists realized that high-risk infants accounted for only about half of infants with hearing loss (Mauk, White, Mortensen, & Behrens, 1991).

Over time, the demand for infant hearing screening has increased significantly. As more premature and critically ill infants survive, the number of infants at risk for hearing loss has also increased and along with it, the need for audiological evaluation of larger numbers of neonates and infants. In 1993, the National Institutes of Health (NIH) organized a Consensus

Conference that resulted in a Consensus Statement (1993) mandating the screening of all infants. Even in light of the NIH mandate, infant screening has not yet become universal. Some hospitals test high-risk children, such as those admitted to the neonatal intensive care unit (NICU) and to neo-natal special care units (NSCU), and those with a known family history of hearing loss. Some hospitals do not routinely test high-risk infants but leave the responsibility of monitoring the hearing of these infants to pediatricians after hospital discharge. Other hospitals routinely screen all infants. In spite of the slow start, it is clear that the hearing of more and more infants is being tested, and the numbers can be expected to increase.

As more infants survive and hearing screening becomes widespread, audiologists will be identifying more infants with hearing loss and will need to learn how to treat them. After diagnosis, the first step in management of hearing loss is the selection and the fitting of appropriate amplification, which requires an accurate assessment of the degree and type of hearing loss, and the obtaining of both ear and frequency-specific information.

Many audiologists feel comfortable testing hearing in infants older than 6 months of age using visual reinforcement audiometry (VRA) but do not feel comfortable testing younger or critically ill infants. However, if an infant fails a hearing screening at birth, we cannot wait until the infant is 6 months old to proceed with diagnosis and habilitation. We must use test techniques that will provide the ear- and frequency-specific information necessary for evaluation, selection, and fitting amplification. Real-ear measures provide good information about how much amplified sound is reaching the ear, but the information is difficult to interpret without good information about the status of the infant's hearing. Tonal auditory brainstem response (ABR) may provide some of this information but it is usually not possible to obtain a complete audiogram using this method, and the thresholds obtained may vary by ±20 dB. Observation audiometry techniques can assist in obtaining the information needed.

Screening Hearing in Neonates

Who Should Be Screened?

Ideally, every infant should be screened for hearing loss and for any other treatable condition that could have an impact on quality or length of life. If that is not possible, audiologists, pediatricians, and neonatologists will be forced to make decisions about who should be screened. As more high-risk infants have been saved and more has become known about the causes of hearing loss in infants, the number of factors listed on the high-risk register has grown, and more neonates have become candidates for hearing testing (American Academy of Pediatrics, 1995; American Speech-Language-Hearing Association [ASHA], 1994). Unfortunately, even if we tested every child who met one or more criteria on the high-risk register, about 50% of children with significant hearing loss would not be identified (Mauk et al). The average age of identification of hearing loss has remained at around 3 years in spite of all efforts to change the situation (Coplan, 1987; Madell and Hoffman, 1987; Parving, 1984; Stein, Clark, & Kraus, 1983; Stein, Jabaley, Spitz, Stoakley, & McGee, 1990). An increased boost to seek early identification of hearing loss was the result of the Healthy People 2000 initiative by Surgeon General C. Everett Koop that sought to reduce the age of identification of hearing-impaired children from 2½ years to 12 months.

It has quickly become clear that universal hearing screening is necessary if we are to identify hearing loss in children in a timely fashion. There has been a great deal of discussion as to exactly when this screening should take place. Some audiologists prefer to give infants and parents time to bond and suggest that hearing screening take place when the infant is 2 to 3 months of age. In fact, Luterman (1997) surveyed parents of hearing-impaired children who reported that they would not want hearing loss identified at birth, preferring to wait until they feel ready to deal with it. Some audiologists suggest waiting until the infant is 6 months of age, when testing is easier to accomplish. Still others do not think universal hearing screening is necessary at all (Bess & Paradise, 1994).

In 1993, the National Institutes of Health (NIH) organized a conference to develop a consensus about infant hearing testing. The NIH Consensus Statement (1993) mandated screening hearing of all infants before hospital discharge and suggested otoacoustic emissions testing (OAE) as the recommended screening protocol. Although there is agreement that there are advantages to waiting to test infants at a few months of age (they are easier to test and parents have had an opportunity to bond with their infant before diagnosis), it is also clear that the neonatal nursery is the only place where audiologists have access to almost all infants. In addition, the Colorado Hearing Project (Apuzzo & Yoshinaga-Itana, 1995) has demonstrated that children who are fitted with amplification and begin habilitation before 6 months of age have an advantage in language development that cannot be made up by those who are fitted later.

Screening of Infants in the Past

NOISEMAKERS

A variety of hearing screening protocols have been used over the years. Noisemakers were the initial test stimulus of choice. A test protocol using noisemakers was developed by the Ewings in England in 1944. Noisemakers were selected because they were readily available, simple and inexpensive, made sounds familiar to the children, could be used in any setting (a soundroom was not required), and were believed to cause infants to respond more reliably than to pure-tone stimuli (Figure 4–1). The difficulty

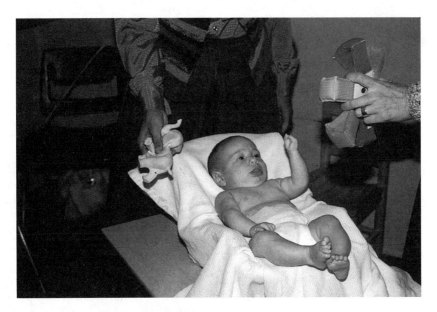

Figure 4–1. Infant testing with noisemakers.

with noisemakers is that they usually have very broad-frequency responses and the intensity is not easy to control, even with practice controlling the pressure used and the distance from the infant's ear. Bove and Flugrath (1973) analyzed 25 noisemakers and concluded that 20 had spectra too broad to be useful. Calibrated signals, such as recorded barking dogs, singing, and train whistles, were also tried, and because they were recorded, the intensity could be controlled. However, the signals were broad-frequency stimuli and responses had to be interpreted with caution.

Even if noisemakers cannot provide information sufficient to be used to assess hearing, they can provide some important gross information about how a child responds to sound. Using noisemakers can tell an audiologist if a child alerts to sound, if she or he can localize the type of response, and the response latency to expect in this particular child. Before using noisemakers, information should be obtained about the auditory signals the noisemakers present, including both the frequency response and intensity. Still, caution must be exercised in how this information is used. Unless the noisemakers have a very narrow frequency range, it is dangerous to make a statement about hearing when using them for screening. For example, a noisemaker may have most of its energy in the 2000 to 4000 Hz range, but have some energy at 500 Hz at 30 to 40 dB less intensity than at the high frequencies. What can we conclude about the infant's response to this stimulus? It is possible that the infant hears the high-frequency component of the stimulus, but it is also possible that the infant has a high-frequency hearing loss, does not hear the high-frequency part of the signal, and is responding to the low-frequency component.

THE HIGH-RISK REGISTER

The high-risk register was first used as a screening tool in 1970 as a result of the work of the Joint Committee on Infant Hearing (ASHA, 1972). Factors known to cause hearing loss were listed, and nurses, physicians, or volunteers reviewed hospital charts and interviewed family members to determine if a child was at risk: a time-consuming activity that required parents to be able to provide reliable information. Parents do not always know enough about family history to provide sufficient information. In addition, half of the children identified with significant congenital hearing loss did not meet any of the high-risk factors and were not identified.

NOISE-GENERATOR HEARING SCREENERS

For infants identified through the high-risk register or by parent or caregiver concern, a technique was needed to screen hearing. A battery-powered instrument was developed that produced a broad-band noise stimulus, usually with high-frequency emphasis. Some instruments presented sounds at several different intensities, usually beginning at 70 dB SPL, others at only one intensity. The tester stood over the infant and directed the megaphone at the infant's ear at a prescribed distance (Figure 4–2).

When possible, testing was done in a quiet room near the nursery, but if no quiet room was available testing was accomplished in the nursery. The protocol involved two observers who stood over the infant and observed responses. Responses included changes in respiration, sucking, limb movements, eye movements, and arousal. Both observers had to agree that a response was present for the response to be accepted. This was clearly a screening test, because no determination could be made about threshold, and frequency-specific information was not available. Any infant for whom there was concern underwent further evaluation.

ABR SCREENING

The logical next choice for infant hearing screening was ABR testing. Audiologists initially used their diagnostic ABR equipment, but when ABR screening became more routine, several manufacturers developed infant-screening devices. The test stimulus is a high-frequency click and identifies hearing loss that is mild to moderate, or worse.

OAE TESTING

With the identification of OAEs by Jack Kemp in 1978, a new technique became available for infant testing. OAE testing is less expensive to perform than ABR, takes less time, and provides more frequency-specific informa-

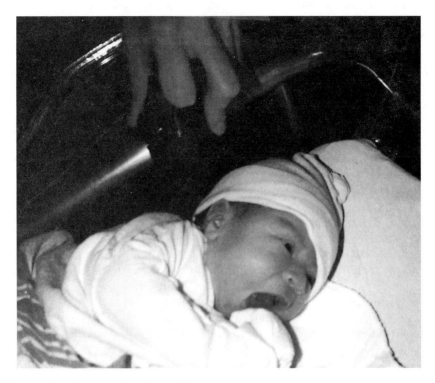

Figure 4–2. Screening hearing with infant screener.

tion, so to some clinicians it seems to be a good choice. Extensive data has been obtained from the Rhode Island Infant Hearing Project (White, Maxon, Behrens, Blackwell, & Vohr, 1992; White, Vohr, & Behrens, 1993) that indicates that OAEs are a reasonable test protocol.

No matter what infant-hearing screening protocol is used, the protocol is only a screening tool. It does not provide sufficient information about hearing to enable the audiologist to fit amplification or provide habilitation without additional information.

Diagnostic Evaluation of Neonates

The goal of the audiological evaluation of an infant is usually to determine if the child has sufficient hearing to develop speech and language. A complete diagnostic evaluation should include immittance testing to assess middle ear status and a test technique to provide frequency and ear-specific information, ideally using both air and bone conduction. The most common test protocols for evaluating neonates include immittance testing and either ABR testing or OAE testing. Immittance testing assesses middle ear status. Niemeyer & Sesterhenn (1972) and Jerger, Burney, & Maudlin (1974) reported a test that looked at the differences in acoustic reflex thresholds to broad-band noise versus pure tones to estimate hearing levels. Information about an infant's ability to hear and to attend to auditory stimuli can only be obtained with behavioral testing, thus no child should be released from follow-up until behavioral test results have been obtained.

Electrophysiological Evaluations

There are two electrophysiological tests routinely used in the evaluation of infants. It is not the purpose of this text to discuss them in detail, but a very brief summary may be useful.

The most frequently used electrophysiological test is ABR. Testing may be accomplished using a broad-band click, or frequency-specific tone pips or noise bursts. Click ABR provides useful information about neurological status, but is not a good choice for a diagnostic hearing evaluation. Because it uses a broad-band stimulus, click ABR may miss an upwardly or a downwardly sloping hearing loss. Frequency-specific ABR testing at 500, 2000, and 4000 Hz in each ear provides sufficient information to rule out anything less than a mild-to-moderate hearing loss. Bone conduction testing can also be accomplished using ABR. Testing requires that the infant sleep for a sufficiently long time to obtain all test results, which may be difficult to accomplish without sedation.

OAE testing provides generalized frequency information but not information about hearing at discrete frequencies. OAEs cannot currently provide threshold information. OAEs will not be present when there is middle ear disease.

Although ABR and OAE testing provide a great deal of information about the functioning of the auditory system, they neither measure hearing nor provide information about the infant's ability to use or to attend to auditory stimuli. Both OAE and ABR testing is difficult to accomplish on a child who is noisy or fussy, or who has neurological disorders. Both systems provide information about the status of the auditory system but not about the infant's or child's ability to use or to attend to auditory information. Such information can only be obtained using behavioral test techniques.

History of Behavioral Evaluation

A variety of behavioral test methods have been used to assess hearing in infants. Because infants (0–6 months) cannot raise their hand or turn their head toward the source of a sound, testing requires observation of an infant's response to the presentation of a sound stimulus.

Attempts were made as early as the 1940s to develop behavioral techniques to assess hearing (Ewing & Ewing, 1940, 1944; Froeschels & Beebe, 1946). Downs & Sterritt (1964, 1967) tried to develop a standardized procedure to assess arousal, but a significant number of false-positive test results made the testing unreliable. Several authors have described techniques for assessing behavioral responses in infants (Beebe, 1951; DiCarlo, Kendell, & Goldstein, 1962; Ewing & Ewing, 1940, 1944; Madell, 1988, 1995). Attempts were made to calibrate the observer so that all observers made the same judgments (Mencher, McCullouch, Derbyshire, & Dethlefs, 1977; Weber, 1969), to assesses the state of the infant (Downs, 1967; Eisenberg, 1969), and calibrate precisely the signal (Moncur, 1968; Thompson & Thompson 1972). In spite of all attempts, observation audiometry continued to be considered "unreliable." Responses obtained were frequently not threshold responses and, as a result, many children failed the test and were identified as hearing impaired when they did not have a hearing loss.

Because the test protocols frequently did not give threshold responses, norms for hearing levels in infants (Northern & Downs, 1984; McConnell & Ward, 1967) considered thresholds of 70 db SPL as normal. Obviously, a child who hears at this level will have significant problems learning language. In fact, more recent reports (Berg & Smith, 1983; Eisele, Berry, & Shriner, 1975; Olsho, 1984; Olsho, et al, 1988; Spenter & Olsho, 1990; Madell, 1995) have demonstrated that infants hear at essentially adult levels. The difficulties in the early work were probably related to test technique, which did not truly measure threshold. By observing the following test protocols, reliable and valid behavioral threshold can be obtained on most neonates and infants.

Observation Audiometry

WHAT ARE WE OBSERVING?

Although many different "behaviors" have been used to assess hearing in infants in the past, (arousal, limb movement, respiration changes, blinking,) they have not proven to be sufficiently repeatable, and more important, have not been good indicators of threshold. My experience indicates that the behavior most likely to provide threshold responses is changes in sucking. Arousal responses, limb movements, and blinking frequently are suprathreshold-level responses, but rarely are threshold responses. Sucking responses, however, are frequently observed at or close to threshold.

MAXIMIZING OBSERVATION OF THE SUCKING RESPONSE

Sucking can be observed with a bottle or with nursing at the breast, or with a pacifier. The family should be instructed to bring the infant to the evaluation hungry so that he or she will be ready to suck. We would like the infant to be as comfortable as possible during testing, so if the infant normally drinks from a bottle, the family should bring one; if the infant normally nurses, it would be best if the infant nursed during testing. For this to succeed, the mother has to be comfortable being observed nursing. It has been my experience that if the mother understands the reason for this intrusion on her privacy, it does not present a problem. If the infant uses a pacifier the family, should bring one along. After the infant has finished eating, testing can frequently continue by observing sucking with a pacifier.

Although we suggest that parents bring in hungry infants for evaluation, it is frequently not possible to test a very hungry baby. If the infant is allowed a little time to eat before beginning to test, she or he will satisfy the initial extreme hunger; as soon as the baby settles down, testing can begin.

EXACTLY WHAT DO WE OBSERVE?

Initiation or cessation of sucking are both acceptable responses. Some infants start sucking when a sound is presented, others cease sucking, and some do both.

HOW DO YOU KNOW THAT THE SUCKING IS IN RESPONSE TO A SOUND STIMULUS?

As with all other behavioral responses, timing is the key factor. When doing play audiometry with a child, we question the validity of a response the child makes if it comes a long time after presentation of the stimulus. As with any test protocol, responses can only be accepted if they occur within a reasonable time after presentation of the stimulus. Each individual infant is fairly consistent. Some respond to the introduction of the stimulus, others respond to its cessation. The timing of the response is also usually consistent. Infants respond at about the same number of seconds after presentation of the stimulus each time. For some infants, the delay is after 1 or 2 seconds, for others it is after 10 seconds.

POSITIONING THE INFANT

The necessity of appropriately positioning the infant cannot be overstated. Indeed, it may be the most important factor in obtaining accurate test results. The infant needs to be seated so as to be visible to the tester, and fully supported, so that the head and the torso are comfortable, not floppy or wobbling. If the infant is nursing (Figure 4–3) the mother holds the child. If the infant is using a bottle or a pacifier she or he may be held (Figure 4–4) or placed in an infant seat (Figure 4–5). An advantage to using an infant seat is that the infant will not receive any "signals" from the mother when she hears the sound. Involuntary movements, such as stiffening by the mother in response to sound, or movement of the breast or bottle, can be transmitted to the infant and influence her or his response to sound. If the infant is being held, the mother or whoever is holding him or her can wear ear-

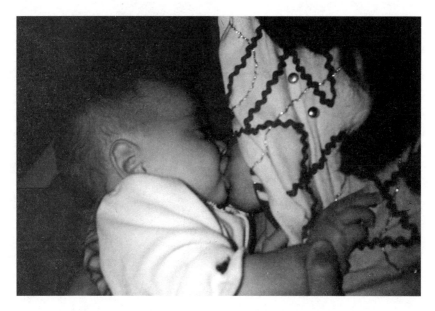

Figure 4–3.   Infant positioned for nursing for observation audiometry.

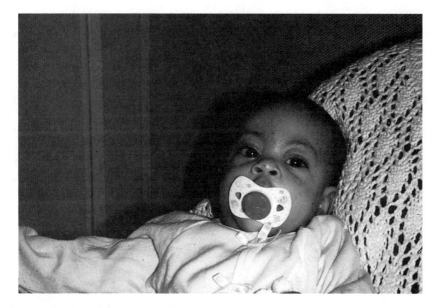

Figure 4–4.   Infant with pacifier for observation audiometry.

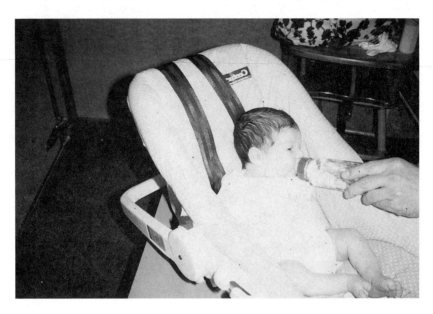

Figure 4–5. Infant positioned in infant seat for observation audiometry.

phones to prevent hearing the sounds and should be carefully instructed about the need to remain silent and still throughout the testing to eliminate interference with test results.

THE ROLE OF THE TEST ASSISTANT

Observation audiometry is best accomplished with two or more observers. One is the audiologist controlling the test equipment, (usually outside of the room in which the infant is placed) and the other is the test assistant, who usually sits next to the infant. Positioning should be carefully done to be certain that both testers can easily see the infant. The test assistant has several responsibilities: The first is constant monitoring of the infant to be certain that the head and the torso are comfortably balanced so that he or she is not fussy or straining. The second is keeping the infant focused at the midline, again so that the she or he is comfortable and not distracted. It may be helpful to hold a colorful toy in front of the infant in a position that allows the infant's head to be centered. Don't hold it above his or her head so that the infant must lift his or her head to see it, or down too low so that the infant bends his or her head down. It is also important that the person holding the toy make no change in its movement when the sound is presented because doing so makes it difficult to determine whether the infant is responding to the sound or to the change in the movement of the toy. Third, the test assistant may also be the one holding the bottle if the child is in an infant seat. Finally, the test assistant will be one of the observers who judges whether or not the infant responded to the sound presentation.

THE ROLE OF THE PARENTS

Parents cannot be relied upon as observers. Their stakes are too high, they are not experienced in the task, and they do not understand exactly what is an acceptable response. However, they are valuable in helping the testers to understand the child and in assisting in making the child comfortable. They should be in the test room so that they understand the test protocols and test results.

Testing Protocol

SOUNDFIELD VERSUS EARPHONE TESTING

The goal of the initial audiological evaluation of an infant is usually to be certain that the infant has sufficient hearing to develop speech and language. As a result, it may not be necessary to obtain ear-specific information at the first visit. Occasionally, an infant is referred for hearing testing because of a medical condition that requires ear-specific information immediately, but this is more frequently the exception than the rule. When it does happen, the test protocol obviously must change. Ear-specific information is important and should be obtained if possible, but the more important question is whether the infant hears enough to learn language. Should the initial evaluation indicate that hearing is normal in at least one ear with soundfield testing, it is not critical immediately to obtain information about each ear separately. However, if the initial testing indicates that hearing is not within normal limits in soundfield, then specific ear information is critical. No infant should be released from follow-up until ear-specific information is obtained.

Under most conditions, testing should begin in soundfield, which provides the important information: Does the child have sufficient hearing to develop speech and language? Earphones (inserts or supra-aural) can be uncomfortable and a distraction to the infant. If the infant is being held for testing, the earphone can become dislodged, altering test results. In addition, infants will only provide a limited number of responses, so testing protocols need to be designed to obtain the most information with the fewest responses. Earphone testing can follow later in the initial test session or at a subsequent test session. When earphone testing is needed, insert earphones are the earphones of choice (Figure 4–6). Supra-aural earphones are frequently too large and are very difficult to keep in place in an infant. On the other hand, insert earphones will remain appropriately seated in the ear canal and provide the most reliable results in tiny ears.

If testing indicates thresholds at less-than-normal hearing levels, bone conduction testing is essential. The bone vibrator should be held in place

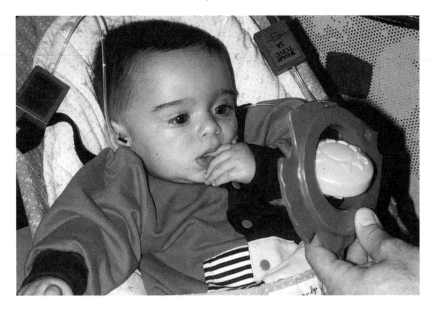

Figure 4–6.   Infant with insert phones.

with a pediatric-sized metal headband (Figure 4–7) or a fabric headband that goes around the head across the forehead using Velcro to secure it (see Figure 4–8). If a metal headband is used, soft material, such as foam or other padding, should be used to keep the headband from moving and digging into the infant's head.

If a hearing loss is confirmed, the same test protocols can be used to assess functional gain with amplification.

TEST STIMULI

When planning testing, it is important to keep in mind that infants will provide only a limited number of responses, so each stimulus presentation must be considered carefully. The goal of the testing is to obtain frequency-specific test results. Warble tones or narrow bands of noise will provide this information. Broad-band stimuli such as music, conversational speech, or white noise will not. Noise bands may provide thresholds that are 5 to 10 dB softer than those obtained with warble tones, but many infants respond more readily to them. The echo test provides an additional stimulus source for infants who are bored with warble tones or noise bands.

Speech-awareness thresholds to low *(ba)*, mid-high *(sh)*, and high *(s)* frequency speech stimuli can be used to confirm warble-tone/noise-band

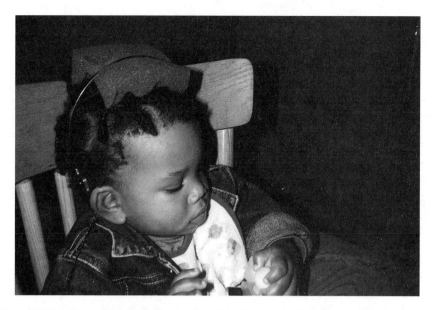

Figure 4–7. Bone vibrator with standard headband.

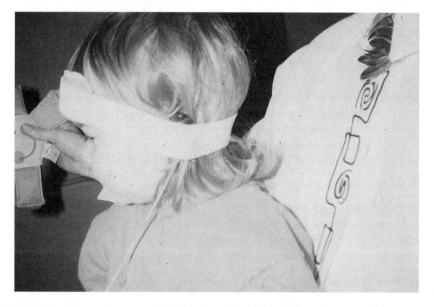

Figure 4–8. Bone vibrator with Velcro headband (made by Huggy, Inc.).

thresholds. The threshold for *ba* should be close (within 10 dB) to the threshold obtained at 500 Hz; *sh* should be close to the threshold obtained at 2000 Hz; and *s* should be close to the threshold obtained at 3000 Hz.

PRESENTATION OF TEST STIMULI

Many infants respond better to low-frequency stimuli, so it is best to begin at a low frequency (usually 500 Hz). If middle ear pathology is a concern, low-frequency hearing may be compromised, so it may be better to begin with a high-frequency stimulus (2000 Hz). After obtaining thresholds at 500 and 2000 Hz, make a determination about what is most important piece of information to have next. If the thresholds at both 500 and 2000 Hz are normal, it is more important to obtain a threshold at 4000 Hz than at 1000 Hz because hearing is likely to also be normal at 1000 Hz. However, if an infant's hearing at 500 Hz is at 30 dB and at 2000 Hz is at 70 dB, it is very important to know what her or his hearing is at 1000 Hz.

Presentation should begin at a level that is loud enough for the infant to hear it, but not so loud as to startle the infant. It is best if the initial stimuli is fairly close to the threshold. If the initial stimulus is much louder than threshold, it may be difficult to get the infant's attention at threshold levels. If an infant has normal hearing, it should be sufficient to begin at 50 to 60 dB. If the infant responds, decrease intensity in 10-dB steps until there is no response, and then increase in 5- or 10-dB steps as you would with any other population. Especially with infants, no response should be recorded until it is observed at the same level 3 times.

Timing is critical. You cannot present stimuli too quickly or the infant will ignore them. A sound that comes out of silence is more likely to get a response. To obtain reliable responses, it is important to observe the infant carefully. The way the infant responds when the stimulus is loud will give you clues about the type and latency of the response that can be expected from the infant as the stimulus intensity decreases.

Adding Objectivity to Observation Audiometry: The Test Setting

INFANT STATE AND POSITIONING

It is important to monitor the infant's state. If the infant moves around a great deal, it will be much more difficult to observe responses. It is essential that the infant be comfortably seated, with head and torso supported, so that nothing interferes with observation of sucking.

MOVEMENT OF TEST ASSISTANT AND PARENT OR CAREGIVER

Everyone in the test room with the child must be still and nonresponsive to the test stimuli, which can be accomplished by having them wear sound-eliminating earphones to prevent them from being aware of the presence of sounds. However, most test assistants and many parents or caregivers can be still and nonresponsive without earphones once they understand the need to do so. The person assigned to keep the infant focused at midline should also be reminded not to respond to the stimulus by altering the movement of the toy or by changing facial expressions.

TEST STIMULI AND RESPONSE

The most critical element for obtaining reliable responses is to predetermine what will constitute a response. If you have decided that sucking is the acceptable response, you should not decide to accept eye-widening or a head turn in the middle of testing because you see something that might be a response. By changing your response criterion during testing, you risk accepting behaviors that are not responses.

The next important criterion is response timing. The response must be time locked to the presentation of the stimulus. It is not reasonable to expect that a response will occur immediately after onset of the stimulus at one presentation and 5 seconds after the stimulus is discontinued a few presentations later. It is not likely that both are responses.

All test stimuli must be repeatable. With infants, responses should be present a minimum of 3 times at the same level before being accepted as a response. Confirming pure-tone/noise-band thresholds with frequency-specific speech stimuli (*ba, sh, s*) will increase reliability.

The use of multiple observers to determine if a response is present also increases reliability, as does the use of silent controls. If the observers are blinded as to the presentation of test stimuli they can be expected to be more "objective" in determining if the infant has made a response. If the observers believe a response is present frequently during silent controls, the reliability of the observers should be questioned.

Test stimuli for infants should be presented with more silent time between stimulus presentations than is common with older children and adults. Presenting test stimuli too close together decreases the likelihood of obtaining many responses because the infant becomes used to the stimulus.

Other Factors Influencing Behavioral Test results with Infants

The audiologist must know something about the infant to obtain reliable test results. Spending a little time with the infant before beginning to test will increase the likelihood of obtaining reliable test results. It is important to have a good estimate of the infant's developmental, neurological, and behavioral status. Can the infant do whatever is required for testing? If we are looking for sucking changes, we need to know that the infant sucks steadily. When an infant has an irregular sucking pattern, it becomes very difficult to observe test responses.

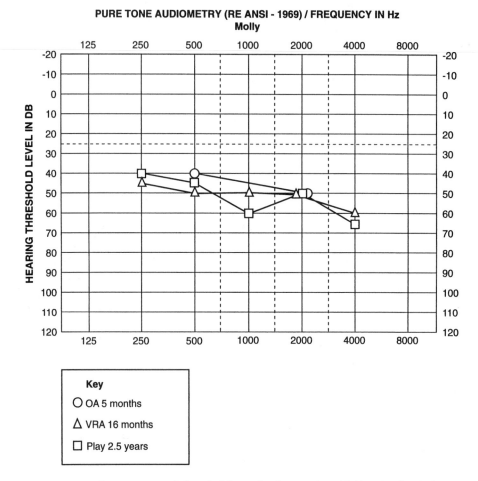

Figure 4–9. Comparison of thresholds with observation (OA), visual reinforcement (VRA), and play audiometry: OA at 5 mo, VRA at 16 mo, Play at 2½ yr.

Are there concerns about the infant's neurological status that could affect testing? For example, is the child alert to the environment? We may be evaluating the infant's hearing, but other aspects of her or his status are important and may influence test results. Is the infant visually alert? Does he or she make postural changes indicating awareness of the presence of people or external stimuli? If the infant is alert to other stimuli but does not respond to sound, this increases the probability that the responses are an indication of a true hearing loss.

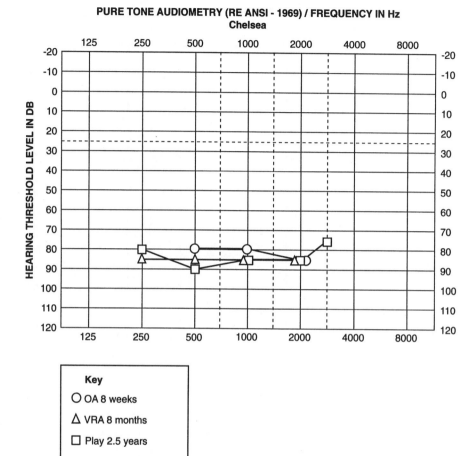

PURE TONE AUDIOMETRY (RE ANSI - 1969) / FREQUENCY IN Hz
Chelsea

Figure 4–10. Comparison of thresholds with observation (OA), visual reinforcement (VRA), and play audiometry: OA at 8 wk, VRA at 8 mo, Play at 2½ yrs.

Comparison of Observation Thresholds to VRA and Play Audiometry

By carefully following test protocols, observation responses can be used to obtain reliable thresholds. Figures 4–9, 4–10, 4–11, and 4–12 are typical of multiple audiograms that demonstrate that thresholds can be obtained accurately using observation audiometry, and they compare thresholds obtained with OA, VRA, and play audiometry over several years on 4 different children. I think they make the best possible case for the reliability of the technique.

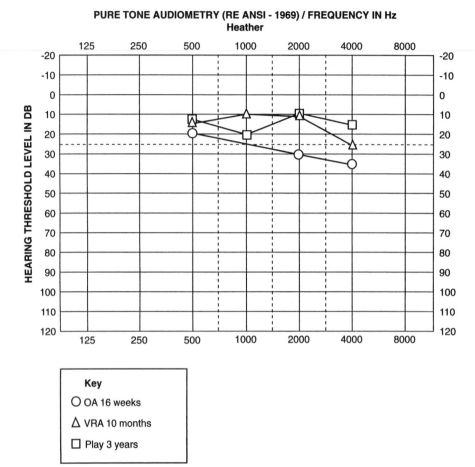

Figure 4–11. Comparison of thresholds with observation (OA), visual reinforcement (VRA), and play audiometry: OA at 16 weeks, VRA at 7 mo, Play at 3 years.

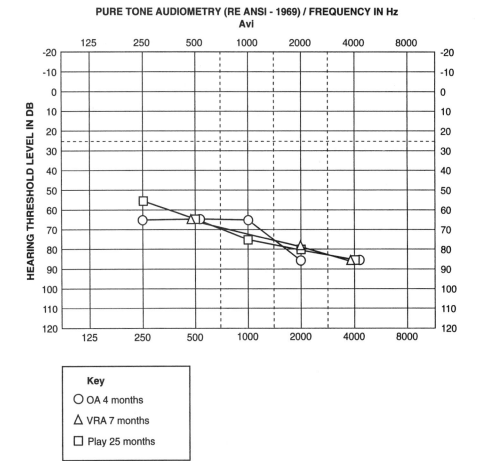

Figure 4–12. Comparison of thresholds with observation (OA), visual reinforcement (VRA), and play audiometry: OA at 4 mo, VRA at 7 mo, Play at 25 mo.

References and Readings

American Academy of Pediatrics. (1995). Joint Committee on Infant Hearing 1994 position statement. *Pediatrics, 95*(1), 152–156.

American Speech-Language-Hearing Association. (1994). Joint Committee on Infant Hearing 1994 position statement, *ASHA, 36*, 38–41.

Apuzzo, M.L., & Yoshinaga-Itana, C. (1995). Early identification of infants with significant hearing loss and the Minnesota Child Development Inventory. *Sem Hear, 16*, 124–139.

Beebe, H.H. (1951). Testing the hearing of young children. *Nervous Child, 9*, 1–14.

Berg, K.M., & Smith, M.C. (1983). Behavioral thresholds of tones during infancy. *J Exp Child Psychol, 35*, 409–425.

Bess, F., & Paradise, J. (1994). Universal screening for infant hearing impairment: Not simple, not risk-free, not necessarily beneficial, and not presently justified. *Pediatrics, 93*, 330–334.

Bove, C., & Flugrath, L. (1973). Frequency components of noisemakers for use in pediatric audiological evaluations. *Volta Rev, 75*, 551–556.

Coplan, J. (1987). Deafness: Ever heard of it? Delayed recognition of permanent hearing loss. *Pediatrics, 79*, 206–212.

DiCarlo, L.M., Kendell, D.C., & Goldstein, R. (1962). Diagnostic procedures for auditory disorders in children. *Folia Phoniatr, 14*, 206–264.

Downs, M.P., & Sterritt, G.M. (1964). Identification audiometry for neonates. A preliminary report. *J of Aud Res, 4*, 69–80.

Downs, M.P., & Sterritt, G.M. (1967). A guide to newborn and infant hearing screening. *Arch Otolaryngol, 85*, 15–22.

Eisele, W.A., Berry, R.C., & Shriner, T.H. (1975). Infant sucking response patterns a conjugate function of change in the sound pressure level of auditory stimuli. *J Speech Hear Res, 18*, 296–307.

Eisenberg, R.B. (1969). Auditory behavior in the human neonate: Functional properties of sound and their ontogenetic implications. *Int Audiology, 8*, 34–45.

Ewing, E.R., & Ewing, A.W.G. (1940). Discussion of audiometric tests and the capacity to hear speech. *J Laryngol Otol, 55*, 339–355.

Ewing, I.R., & Ewing, A.W.F. (1944). The ascertainment of deafness in infancy and early childhood. *J Laryngol Otol, 59*:309–333.

Froding, C.A. (1960). Acoustic investigation of newborn infants. *Acta Otolaryngol, 52*, 31–41.

Froeschels, E., & Beebe, H. (1946). Testing the hearing of the newborn. *Arch Otolaryngol, 44*, 710–714.

Jerger, J., Burney, P., & Maudlin, L. (1974). Predicting hearing loss from the acoustic reflex *J Speech Hear Disord, 39*, 11–22.

Kemp, D.T. (1978). Stimulated acoustic emissions from within the human auditory system. *J Acoust Soc Am, 64*, 1386–1391.

Luterman, D. (1997). Counseling parents of hearing impaired children. Paper presented at the American Academy of Audiology Annual Convention, April 17–20, Fort Lauderdale, FL.

Madell, J.R. (1988). Identification and treatment of very young children with hearing loss. *Infants Young Children, 1*, 20–30.

Madell, J.R. (1995). Behavioral evaluation of infants after hearing screening: Can it be done? *Hear Instruments, 12*, 4–8.

Madell, J.R., & Hoffman, R.A. (1987). Delay in pediatric referral for audiologic evaluation. Paper presented at the American Speech-Language-Hearing (ASHA) Convention, November, Chicago, IL.

Mauk, G.A., White, K.R., Mortensen, L.B., & Behrens, T.R. (1991). The effectiveness of screening programs based on high-risk characteristics in early identification of hearing impairment. *Ear Hear, 12*, 312–318.

McConnell, F., & Ward, P. (1967). *Deafness in Childhood*. Nashville: Vanderbilt University Press.

Mencher, G.T., McCullouch, B., Derbyshire, A.J., & Dethlefs, R. (1977). Observer bias as a factor in neonatal hearing screening. *J Speech Hear Res, 20*, 27–34.

Moncur, J. (1968). Judge reliability in infant testing. *J Speech Hear Res, 11*, 348–357.

National Institutes of Health. (1993). Consensus statement: Early identification of hearing impairment in infants and young children. March 1–3, 1993, Bethesda, MD.

Niemeyer, W., & Sesterhenn, G. (1972). Calculating the hearing threshold from the stapedius reflex threshold for different sound stimuli. *J Aud Commun, 11,* 84.

Northern, J., & Downs, M. (1984). *Hearing in Children* (3rd ed.). Baltimore: Williams & Wilkins.

Olsho, L.W. (1984). Infant frequency discrimination. *Infant Behav Dev, 7,* 27–35.

Olsho, L.W., Koch, E., Carter, E., Halpin, C., & Spenter, N. (1988). Pure-tone sensitivity of human infants. *J Acoustical Society of North America, 84,* 1316–1324.

Parving, A. (1984). Early detection and identification of congenital/early acquired disability. Who takes the initiative? *Int J Ped Otorhinolaryngol, 7,* 107–117.

Spenter, N.B., & Olsho, L.W. (1990). Auditory frequency resolution in human infancy. *Child Devp, 61,* 632–652.

Stein, L., Clark, S., & Kraus, N. (1983). The hearing-impaired infant: Patterns of identification and habilitation. *Ear Hear, 4,* 232–236.

Stein, L., Jabaley, T., Spitz, R., Stoakley, D., & McGee, T. (1990). The hearing-impaired infant: patterns of identification and habilitation revisited. *Ear Hear, 11,* 201–205.

Thompson, M., & Thompson, F. (1972). Response of infants and young children as a function of auditory stimuli and test method. *J Speech Hear Res, 15,* 699–707.

U.S. Department of Health and Human Services, Public Health Service. (1990). *Healthy People 2000: National Health Promotion and Disease Prevention Objectives.* Washington, D.C.: U.S. Government Printing Office.

Weber, B.A. (1969). Validation of observer judgements in behavioral observation audiometry. *J Speech Hear Res, 34,* 350–356.

Wedenberg, E. (1956). Auditory tests on newborn infants. *Acta Otolaryngol, 46,* 446–461.

Werner, L., & Gillenwater, J. (1990). Pure tone sensitivity of 2–5 week old infants. *Infant Behav Dev, 13,* 355–375.

White, K.R., Maxon, A.B., Behrens, T.B., Blackwell, P.M., & Vohr, B.R. (1992). Neonatal screening using evoked otoacoustic emissions: The Rhode Island hearing assessment project. In Bess, F.H., & Hall, J.W. III (eds.): *Screening Children for Auditory Function.* Nashville: Bill Wilkerson Center Press.

White, K.R., Vohr, B.R., & Behrens, T.B. (1993). Universal newborn screening using transient evoked otoacoustic emissions: Results of the Rhode Island hearing assessment project. *Semin Hear, 14,* 18–29.

5

Visual Reinforcement Audiometry: Testing Infants from 6 to 36 Months

Behavioral methods are the first choice for diagnostic testing of auditory function because they provide the most information about an infant's ability to hear. Once infants reach between 5 and 6 months, behavioral testing becomes much easier to accomplish because infants can be conditioned to respond to sound. The most common test techniques involve training the infant to make a conditioned head turn in response to a test stimulus. Infants only a few months old will naturally turn toward a sound source. Most infants turn toward the sound source a few times, but the head-turning behavior will habituate to repeated stimuli. Fortunately, head-turning behavior can be shaped, using an operant discrimination procedure to obtain numerous responses to auditory stimuli. The sound stimulus is used to cue the infant to seek the reinforcement. Use of a positive reinforcement, such as a lighted toy, increases the number of responses. Conditioned responses have the advantage of being more repeatable than those obtained in observation audiometry, and more responses can usually be obtained during one session. A number of conditioned techniques have been used. Visual reinforcement audiometry ([VRA] Liden & Kankkunen, 1969) and conditioned orienting response audiometry ([COR] Suzuki & Ogiba, 1960) are the techniques most commonly used. VRA uses a conditioned head turn reinforced by a lighted toy. COR requires that the infant find the sound source before reinforcement with a lighted toy, and reinforcement is only provided if the child turns to the correct side. Visually reinforced operant conditioned response (VROCA) and tangible reinforced operant conditioned audiometry (TROCA) are used less frequently, but have been found to be valuable for certain populations.

TROCA provides a tangible reinforcer (e.g., food) to encourage the infant to respond.

Visual Reinforcement Audiometry

The foundation for VRA was laid by Suzuki and Ogiba in work published in 1960; the name was first used by Liden and Kankkunen in 1969. The technique was refined by Moore, Wilson, and Thompson in numerous publications between 1977 and 1984. VRA is the most commonly used of the reinforcement procedures and is the one discussed in this chapter. It is used to evaluate hearing in children who are cognitively between 5 to 6 and 36 months old. It uses a conditioned head-turning response that is shaped by the examiner's control of a stimulus–reinforcement paradigm. The audiologist presents a stimulus; if the child detects the stimulus, she or he turns toward the stimulus. The audiologist then activates a reinforcer. After a few repetitions, the child learns to seek the reinforcer when he or she hears the sound (Primus & Thompson, 1987).

VRA can be performed using loudspeakers, earphones, a bone conduction vibrator, or hearing aids. For sound field testing, the test room needs to be large enough to have loudspeakers set up at a sufficient distance from the infant to permit a sufficient head turn. If the room is too small, the loudspeakers and reinforcing toy may be within the child's line of sight when she or he is facing forward. Since the response we are seeking is a conditioned head turn, the child should be seated at no less than a 45° angle from the loudspeakers and reinforcer, and preferably at 90°. The toy should not be in the child's line of sight when he or she is facing forward. The test setup needs to be such that there is no doubt as to whether or not the infant made a head turn rather than gave a casual gaze toward the toy.

Ideally, the child should be seated in a highchair and not on a parent's lap (Figure 5–1). If the child is on an adult's lap, the adult may respond to the sound and inadvertently give a cue to the infant. If the child must sit on an adult's lap, the adult needs to be instructed not to respond in any way to the presentation of the sound stimulus. If there is any doubt about the adult's ability to sit still during the test session, she or he can wear noise-canceling earphones to reduce the chance of responding to the stimulus. However, the use of earphones may make it difficult for the adult to interact with the infant, which may make the infant uncomfortable.

Accurate VRA depends on the ability of the examiner or test assistant to keep the child attentive. An audiologist, test assistant, or parent needs to be

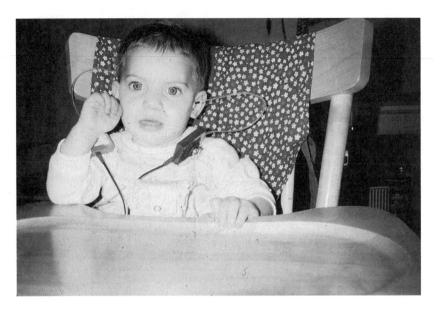

Figure 5–1. Child seated in highchair for VRA testing.

responsible for keeping the infant facing forward. Using colorful toys, puppets, finger games, or making funny faces will keep the infant focused straight ahead so that a clear head turn can be observed. The test room should not be cluttered. Toys that are not being used should be out of sight so that the infant will not be distracted from the adult who is keeping the child focused.

Visual Reinforcers

A variety of toys are available for use as reinforcers. Moore, Thompson, and Thompson (1975) investigated the use of different reinforcers and their effect on responses. They compared no reinforcement, social reinforcement, blinking lights, and complex visual reinforcement, and concluded that complex reinforcement resulted in significantly more localizations than did simple reinforcers. The best reinforcers are novel and interesting. Mechanical toys that are brightly illuminated are excellent (Figure 5–2, and Figure 5–3). A variety is available, including clowns that play drums, dogs that bark, and elephants that eat ice cream cones. Ideally, the reinforcer should be enclosed in a cloudy Lucite™ box so the toy is not easily observable until it is turned on. Most systems permit turning

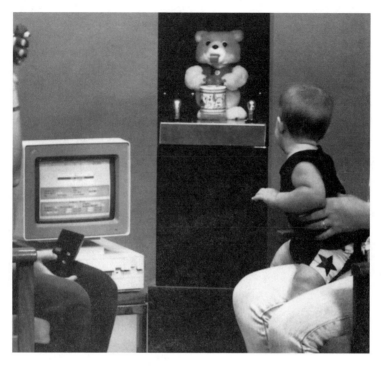

Figure 5–2.   VRA toys. (Photo courtesy of IVRA.)

on the sound and lights either separately or together. This is particularly useful when a child is frightened by the noise made by the reinforcing toy.

For older children, a cartoon video works particularly well as a reinforcer. The television (TV) sound should be off so that it does not to interfere with test stimuli. Because the video constantly changes, it will be of ongoing interest. A small TV with videocassette recorder (VCR) can be placed above the speaker and turned on and off like the mechanical toy.

Occasionally, children react negatively to the reinforcers. Some children are frightened by the sound or the movement. If the sound creates a problem, it can be turned off and the lights can be used alone. If the movement is a problem, the toy can be held still and a light on the toy can be flashed on and off as a reinforcer. If the child is disturbed by the toys regardless of whether they are making noise or moving, an alternative method is to darken the tester's room and shine a flashlight into the test room through the test-room window as a reinforcer. The light can either flash on and off

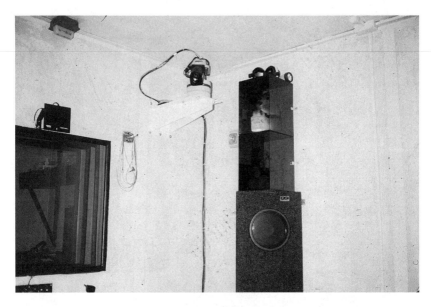

Figure 5–3. VRA toys.

or can be waved around. A head turn towards the tester's window determines a response.

Positioning the Infant or Child

A critical factor in obtaining reliable VRA thresholds is keeping the infant's or child's attention focused at midline in a position that easily permits a head turn. Proper positioning is essential. The child needs to be seated comfortably so that the upper body is steady, allowing the infant or child to turn easily to look at the toy. He or she should not be leaning over trying to get something from the floor, trying to maintain balance, or looking for something or someone seated behind. Older children with very good body control may be able to make a head turn of 180° to look for the reinforcer, but a young or neurologically impaired child will not be able to do so. For these children, a head turn of more than 90° is very difficult and may significantly reduce the ability to respond, so it is critical that these children be focused carefully at midline.

If the infant does not yet have good upper body control due to age, or to a neurological or developmental disorder, and falls when left in a sitting position, it will be difficult for her or him to make a head-turn response. Correct positioning for these children is especially important. An infant without good upper body control should be seated leaning back in a reclining seat or against a parent so that he or she does not have to struggle to maintain position and has enough energy to make a head turn toward the reinforcer.

Distractors

Someone needs to be responsible for keeping the infant focused at midline. If there is a test assistant, this is his or her job. Parents or caregivers are often very good at this task. With limited instruction they can frequently do this job very well, especially with normally developing children. They know their children well and know how to entertain them. If a parent is to have the responsibility of distracting the child, he or she needs to be told to be relatively quiet so as not to interfere with presentation of test stimuli. Even more critical, she or he must be told not to react to the sound in any way, which might provide a cue to the child. Instructions should include acting "deaf" to the sound and not: (a) looking up when the sound goes on to see the child's response; (b) looking at the reinforcement toy until *after* the child does; (c) changing body language when the sound is presented; or (d) altering the way the toys are being played with when the sound is presented.

A variety of toys can be useful as distractors; they should be quiet, simple, and interesting but not engrossing. Young children should view the toys being manipulated by the test assistant but should not handle them because it will probably be too distracting. Older children may be able to manipulate certain toys as long as the toys are not too interesting or require too much concentration. Edible distractions are frequently very useful, provided they are not too noisy. (e.g., crunchy food interferes with listening.)

Training the Response

There are two approaches to training the response. The first is to pair the stimulus with the reinforcer, and the second is to begin by observing the response and then providing a reinforcer. During the initial training trials, it is essential that the audiologist be certain that the infant hears the sound before activating the reinforcer. If the reinforcer is activated when there is no stimulus or when the infant cannot hear the stimulus, he or she will not be able to make the association between the sound and the reinforcer, and will be confused. If there is any question at all about whether or not the infant heard the stimulus, the reinforcer should not be activated. A good rule: *if in doubt, don't.* You lose nothing by failing to reinforce when a stimulus is present, but you may lose a great deal by reinforcing when the infant has not heard a stimulus.

If a child has anything less than a severe or profound hearing loss, it should be relatively easy to get an initial response. The child should be seated in the high chair or on a parent's lap, facing forward. The room does not need to be silent, but it should be relatively quiet. The audiologist begins by presenting stimuli at a level at which the child is expected to respond. If the child hears the sound she or he will probably look up from the toy and search for the sound source. If there is no response, the audiologist increases the intensity until there is a response. Once a response has been obtained, the reinforcer is turned on. If the infant looks up but does not turn to the reinforcer, the parent or test assistant should attract the child's attention to the reinforcer. When this has been done a few times, the infant will have learned the task and testing can begin. Before attracting the child's attention to the reinforcer it is *essential* that the audiologist be absolutely certain that the child has heard the sound.

Children with significant hearing losses or with auditory attention or auditory processing problems may not be able to locate the sound. For these children, in particular, it is necessary to pair the stimulus with the sound and to teach the child to seek the reinforcer. If the infant does not respond to even very loud sounds, it may be useful to try to train her or him to a tactile stimulus. Place a bone vibrator in the infant's hand and have the test assistant or parent hold it in place. Even a child with no usable hearing will be able to feel the bone vibrator. The sound is then paired with the reinforcer, thus conditioning the child to that stimulus. After the child has responded consistently to a tactile stimulus, return to an air-conducted stimulus in sound field or under earphones and try the test again. If the reason for lack of response is the severity of the hearing loss, it is essential that the infant accept earphones because earphone signals can almost always be presented at a higher intensity than those from loudspeakers.

The intensity of the initial test stimuli is important. Ideally, the stimulus should be presented slightly, but not too much, above threshold. Several researchers (Eilers, Miskiel, Ozdamar, Urbano, & Widen, 1991, a,b; Tharp & Ashmead, 1993) have demonstrated that the starting level influences false responses. The higher the starting intensity, the greater the false-response rate.

Frequency of Reinforcing the Response

The tendency of most testers is to reinforce every response the child makes, which causes two problems. First, the anxiety to provide a reinforcement occasionally causes the audiologist to reinforce when the infant has not really provided a head turn, confusing the infant and reducing response reliability. Second, frequent reinforcement causes more rapid habituation to the response. Research on behavioral conditioning has demonstrated that intermittent reinforcement is more reliable than constant reinforcement and provides more responses. The best reinforcement schedule begins with 100% reinforcement and decreases to less-frequent reinforcement. Occasionally failing to reinforce the response increases the total number of responses the infant is likely to provide during a test session.

Test Stimuli

Any test stimulus used in behavioral testing can be used with VRA. Speech stimuli are frequently used as the initial test stimulus with children because speech stimuli are familiar and are likely to get the attention of the child. Any speech stimulus can be used to obtain a speech awareness threshold. To obtain frequency-specific speech information, it is necessary to use low, mid-high, and high-frequency stimuli (such as *ba, sh,* and *s*) rather than a broad-band stimulus such as music, or running speech (e.g., *"Hello, Jody. How are you today?"*). These frequency-specific speech thresholds should provide thresholds that are in agreement with pure tone thresholds at low, mid-high, and high frequencies. This will not be true of broad-band speech stimuli, which are in agreement with the softest pure-tone threshold. (See Chapter 9 for more information about speech audiometry with children.)

To obtain a complete audiogram, we obviously need thresholds at several, if not all, frequencies. Although pure tones are usually the stimuli of choice, others are also very useful and may be helpful in obtaining a complete audiogram. Narrow bands of noise may be more interesting to infants and young children and may hold their attention better than pure tones. Alternating between pure tones and noise bands may also increase interest and the number of repeatable responses. Noise bands provide thresholds 5 to 10 dB softer than those obtained with pure tones, which should be taken into consideration when evaluating the responses. For soundfield testing, warbled pure tones are the stimuli of choice because pure tones can create standing waves that reflect off the sound room walls, resulting in invalid threshold levels. As with earphone testing, noise bands are a good second stimulus.

Test Conditions

The use of VRA is reliable in all test conditions required for the evaluation of hearing in infants and young children. Testing can be accomplished in soundfield, with standard supra-aural earphones (see Figure 5–4), insert earphones, a bone vibrator, and amplification, allowing us to obtain almost any audiological information we need.

Test Protocol

Some audiologists begin every evaluation with immittance testing. Although there is no doubt about the usefulness of this procedure, it is important to take the child into consideration when selecting tests and test order. An infant who is frightened of the test facility or of the tester may become

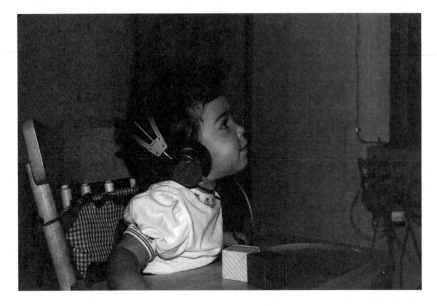

Figure 5–4. Child with headphones seated for VRA.

distressed by having a stranger place an immittance probe in the ear at the beginning of the evaluation. If you proceed with the test and the child becomes upset, the rest of the testing may be difficult or impossible to accomplish. If the child seems distressed or even wary at the outset, it may be better to wait until the end of the session for immittance testing.

The same case can be made for the decision as to whether to begin testing using earphones or loudspeakers. There is no doubt that earphone testing is the goal, but it may be better to get some information in sound field before presenting earphones. When testing very young children, it is useful to assume that each response obtained may be the last, so it is important to think carefully about the order of testing. If you use earphones first and the child becomes upset and gives only one reliable response, you will not have much information. However, if you can keep the child happy, start in soundfield, and obtain thresholds at 500 and 2000 Hz, you will be able to provide some information about the child's hearing, even if you have to stop there.

Most pediatric audiologists begin by using speech audiometry. It is familiar and usually easily gains the attention of an infant or a young child, especially if the test room is quiet. The most useful speech stimuli are frequency-specific stimuli (*ba, sh, s*) because they provide information about the contour of the audiogram and confirm pure-tone/noise-band thresholds. After speech-awareness thresholds have been obtained, providing a general picture of the child's hearing, frequency-specific thresholds should be obtained using a combination of noise bands and warbled pure tones.

If there is concern about middle ear pathology, low-frequency hearing may be poorer than high-frequency hearing. In this case, it is best to begin with a high frequency (2000 Hz), which should be more easily heard. Once a threshold has been obtained at 2000 Hz, proceed to 500 Hz. If the child is speech- and language-delayed, and there is concern about a possible sensorineural hearing loss, low frequencies are likely to be better heard than high frequencies, so testing should begin at 500 Hz.

Applying the theory that each threshold obtained may be the last requires good planning when testing. After beginning to test at 500 or 2000 Hz (depending on whether there is concern about conductive or sensorineural hearing loss), a decision must be made about how to proceed. Depending on the contour of the partial audiogram and the cooperativeness of the child, decide if it would be better to test at 4000 Hz, 500 Hz, or 250 Hz, or with a bone conduction transducer or earphones. If the audiogram is sloping downward, testing at 4000 Hz is important; if upward, there is a good chance the loss is conductive, and testing with a bone conduction transducer might be next. If the audiogram is flat, indicating a hearing loss, earphone testing may be the procedure of choice to obtain separate ear information. If it is not possible to obtain bone conduction thresholds, immittance may provide sufficient information to begin to plan treatment.

Getting a young child to wear earphones can be tricky but is usually possible. Start by having the test assistant wear the earphones, then the parents, then offer them to the child. If she or he refuses, give everyone else a chance to wear the earphones again, and then, offer them again to the child. If the child still refuses, you must make a judgment about how serious the refusal is. If you feel the protest is minimal, try pushing the matter: Have one person keep the child occupied with a toy while another puts the earphones on the child. Frequently, once the child hears a sound and sees the reinforcer, the resistance stops or, at least, decreases to a level that permits testing to proceed. If this method doesn't work, and the child starts to become upset, it may be better to stop and try again at a later date, try different earphones (inserts versus supra-aural), or try a hand-held supra-aural earphone at the child's ear. Supra-aural earphones are easy to put on and frequently can be put in place in a few seconds. However, they can be heavy for an infant's head, making it difficult for her or him to turn toward the reinforcer, and the earphones can fall off with movement. Insert earphones are more comfortable to wear because they are lightweight, but they require more effort to put in the ear.

If you do get the child to wear the earphones, you are again faced with the decision of what to test. Again, assume that each response may be the last. The first goal is to obtain thresholds at 500 Hz and 2000 Hz in each ear, and then fill in, as needed. If there is concern about conducive hearing loss, begin with 2000 Hz in each ear and then change to 500 Hz. If there is concern related to sensorineural hearing loss, begin at 500 Hz, then increase to 2000 Hz. Next, proceed to 4000 Hz, 500 Hz, or 250 Hz, depending on the contour of the audiogram. The 1000-Hz threshold may be left to last; this threshold often is not tested because it can frequently be estimated from the other thresholds. However, if there is a significant difference between the thresholds at 500 and 2000 Hz, it is critical to test at 1000 Hz before proceeding to other frequencies to get a good picture of the audiometric contour.

If testing is performed using earphones, loudspeakers, and bone conduction transducers, consider testing different frequencies with each transducer. The combination of all will provide a fairly complete picture of the child's hearing (Figure 5–5).

When testing children, audiologists frequently feel they must obtain many responses before recording thresholds. This is understandable, but doing so may significantly reduce the number of thresholds obtained. Infants and young children only respond for a limited time, so each stimulus presentation must be carefully considered. Eilers, et al (1991 a and b) used computer simulation to test infants and determined that more than three reversals were not useful in obtaining thresholds: there was less than a 3-dB difference when more than three reversals were obtained, so trust the response you are observing.

Audiologists frequently make a mistake related to the timing of presentation of the stimulus when testing young children. Because we are in a hurry when testing infants, knowing that we may not get many responses, we frequently present stimuli too quickly. If a child is asked to make a conditioned head turn frequently, both the stimulus and the reinforcer become uninteresting, and the child will stop responding. Taking time and presenting stimuli after a longer period of silence increases the likelihood that the stimulus will be interesting and cause the child to look up. On the other hand, having an extended "off" period can also have a negative effect and cause the child to tune out. The correct timing varies from child to child.

There has been much discussion about what is considered normal hearing in infants. Early data (Northern & Downs, 1984; Primus & Thompson, 1991) indicated that normally hearing infants did not respond to sound until it reached a level of about 60 db HL. Recent work (Diefendorf & Gravel, 1996; Madell, 1995) has demonstrated that infants with normal hearing respond to sound that is at only slightly higher than that at adult levels. Infant response should be at no more than 15 db HL.

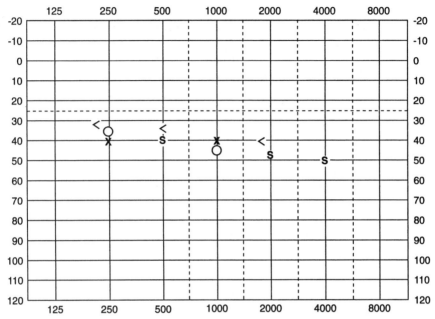

PURE TONE AUDIOMETRY (RE ANSI - 1969)
FREQUENCY IN Hz

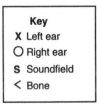

Key
X Left ear
O Right ear
S Soundfield
< Bone

Figure 5–5. Audiogram obtained using different transducers at different frequencies (soundfield, earphones, and bone vibrator).

Factors that Effect Test Results

Several factors affect the reliability of the test results: *Developmental age* is critical. As we have said, it is essential to know the child's developmental age to select the appropriate test protocol. *Neurological status* is also critical. The child must be capable of attending and of making the appropriate physical response (in this case, a conditioned head turn.) If the child's neurological status does not permit a head turn, the test will not be valid. *Be-*

havioral status is also important. If a child is fussy or uncomfortable, you may not get the best results. It may be worth taking the time to make her or him comfortable, (change diapers, provide food and comfort) before proceeding with the test. *Positioning* is very important. If the infant is seated in a way that reduces upper-body control, there is little chance that he or she will be able to make reliable, conditioned head turns. If neurological development is delayed, the range of the required head turn must be limited. Requiring a head turn of more than 90° will not likely be successful. *Distractors* must be engaging but not engrossing, and *reinforcers* must be interesting and attractive. The *test stimuli* should be varied to keep the child's attention, and *presentation timing* should be varied enough to be unpredictable.

For a new tester, this all may sound like a great deal to keep in mind, and initially, it is. But with experience, it becomes second nature. However, during any hearing evaluation, even the most experienced tester should stop when test problems arise, review what he or she is doing, and think about what might be done to improve test results.

References and Readings

Eilers, R.E., Miskiel, E., Ozdamar, O., Urbano, R., & Widen, J.E. (1991a). Optimization of automated hearing test algorithms: Simulations using an infant response model. *Ear Hear, 12,* 191–198.

Eilers, R.E., Widen, J.E., Urbano, R., Hudson, T.M., & Gonzales, L. (1991b). Optimization of automated hearing test algorithms: A comparison of data from stimulations and young children. *Ear Hear, 12,* 199–204.

Liden, G., & Kankkunen, A. (1969). Visual reinforcement audiometry. *Acta otolaryngol, 67,* 281–292.

Madell, J. (1995). Behavioral evaluation of infants after hearing screening: Can it be done? *Hearing Instruments, 12,* 4–8.

Moore, J.M., Thompson, G., & Thompson, M. (1975). Auditory localization of infants as a function of reinforcement conditions. *J Speech Hear Disord, 40* 29–34.

Moore, J.M., Wilson, W.R., & Thompson, G. (1977). Visual reinforcement of head-turn responses in infants under 12 months of age. *J Speech Hear Disord, 42,* 328–334.

Northern, J., & Downs, M. (1984). *Hearing in Children.* Baltimore: Williams and Wilkins.

Primus, M.A. (1991). Repeated infant thresholds in operant and nonapparent audiometric procedures. *Ear Hear, 12,* 119–122.

Primus, M.A., & Thompson, G. (1985). Response strength of young children in operant audiometry. *J Speech Hear Res, 28,* 539–547.

Suzuki, T., & Ogiba, Y. (1960). A technique of pure-tone audiometry for children under three years of age: Conditioned orientation reflex (COR) audiometry. *Rev Laryngol Otol Rhinol, 81,* 33–45.

Tharp, A.M., & Ashmead, D.H. (1993). Computer simulation technique for assessing pediatric auditory test protocols. *J Am Acad Audiol, 4,* 80–90.

6

Play Audiometry:
Testing Children 2½ Years and Older

Once children reach a cognitive age of about 30 months, they can begin voluntarily to cooperate in hearing testing. By this age, children can be taught to drop a toy in a bucket or put a ring on a ring stand when they hear a sound (Figures 6–1, 6–2). This development is both positive and negative. If we can get the child's cooperation we can learn a great deal about the child's hearing, but if we cannot, we may not learn anything about his or her hearing. The challenge for the audiologist is to find ways to keep the young child entertained for a long enough time to complete the hearing test.

Assessing the Child's Cognitive Age

As with all other behavioral test techniques, the first task is to determine the child's cognitive age. Regardless of the child's chronological age, behavioral testing requires that we know the child's cognitive age. Play audiometry is easily accomplished with children who are cognitively older than 3 years of age but not with children under 2½ years. Some children are able to perform play tasks at about 2 years, but many are not, and those who can do so may not be able to perform the task long enough to complete an audiogram. Selecting the wrong test procedure means that the audiologist may obtain no thresholds, few thresholds, or inaccurate thresholds.

Cognitive information can be obtained in a number of ways. A good history of the child will provide some information. If the child's motor development is within normal limits and he or she has no other significant developmental issues (e.g., autism or pervasive developmental disorder

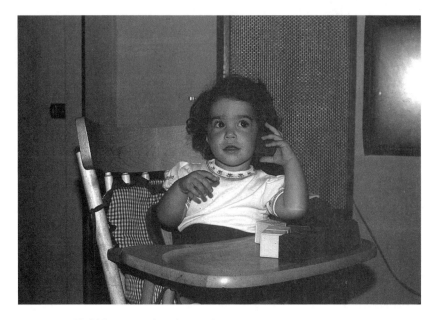

Figure 6–1. Child listening for play audiometry.

[PDD]), you can expect the child to be able to perform the play task. If speech and language development are grossly within normal limits as determined by observation, cognitive levels can be assumed to be close to normal. If a child has other developmental disabilities, cognitive levels will be harder to ascertain and the results of developmental tests may be required. Once you have determined that a child is cognitively older than 30 months, play audiometry can be attempted. Children who have frequent hearing tests, such as those with hearing loss or recurrent otitis media, are likely to learn play earlier. Visual reinforcement audiometry (VRA) may become boring for these children after repeated testing, and once they are familiar with the audiologist and the test environment, they may be willing to try the play task.

Training a Child for Play Audiometry

When conditioning a child to play audiometry, it is critical to know for certain that the child has heard the sound we are using to train the response. (If the child has not heard the sound, we will be conditioning them to silence and confusing the child.) After having taken a history and interacted with the child during the interview, the audiologist should have an idea about where to begin. If the child responds to conversation, you can proba-

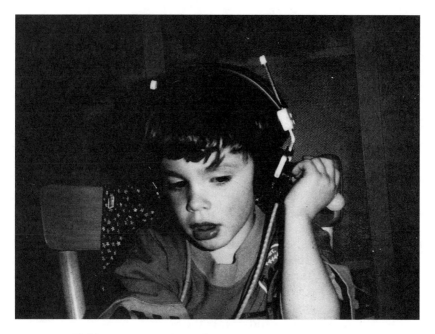

Figure 6–2. Child wearing earphones listening for play audiometry.

bly begin by presenting test stimuli at 30 to 40 dB. If the child does not respond to conversation but seems to be developing normally in other ways (motor development, play activities) it is possible that the child has a significant hearing loss and a loud stimulus will be needed to condition the child.

Training the Task

The play audiometry task requires that the child hold a toy up to his or her ear and perform a motor task (e.g., drop the toy in the bucket) when the sound is presented. The toy is held up to the ear as a signal that the child is ready to listen and so that the motor act of dropping the toy in the bucket is clear. If the child is playing with the toy, or holding it right above the bucket, and drops it in, it is not clear whether it was truly a response to the sound or a decision the child made at that moment. When training the child for the task, begin with an easy play activity, such as dropping a block in a bucket, not one that requires dexterity, such as fitting a chip into a slot or a small peg into a hole.

There are several ways to begin. The test assistant can begin by demonstrating the task, holding the toy to her or his ear, and when the sound is presented saying, "I hear that," and dropping the toy into the bucket. If the child seems hesitant, allow the parent to try for one or two sound presentations. Then, hand the child the toy, hold his or her hand up to his or her ear, and when the sound is presented say, "We heard that," and moving his or her hand, drop the toy in the bucket. After one or two tries, let the child do it alone. If the child seems hesitant and you are certain that she or he has heard the sound, give the child's hand a nudge to help her or him to begin. If the child still needs assistance, try demonstrating the task again saying, "Okay, it's my turn." You can also try to do it together, with both the tester and the child holding toys and dropping them in the bucket when the sound is presented. You must be careful that the child is not simply imitating your motor task, or dropping the block when you do, but is actually responding to a sound stimulus.

After several training attempts, the child must do it alone. Say, "It's your turn," and let the child begin the task. If the child looks up when the sound is presented but is hesitant about putting the toy in the bucket, you can say, "You heard that, put it in." If the child continues to look to you for approval before putting the toy in, try looking away at the floor, or at the bucket to signal to the child that she or he is on her own. If the child is still unable to do the task, start over again and retrain the task.

If you are uncertain if the child has heard the sound, even at loud levels, try conditioning the child with the bone vibrator from the audiometer. Even a child with no hearing will feel the tactile response of the bone vibrator at 250 Hz. Place the vibrator in the child's hand and hold his hand closed with your own. Use your other hand to help the child hold the toy up to his or her ear and place it in the bucket when the vibrator is turned on. Once the child has learned the task with the vibrator, return to an air-conducted stimulus and try again.

Test Protocol

Choosing the Test Stimulus

If a child responds to speech (e.g., answering when called) you may want to begin with a speech stimulus. The easiest may be the command, "Put it in." The child will understand the verbal command and learn the task easily, which will provide you with a speech-awareness threshold but will not frequency-specific information. Once the child has been conditioned to the task, change the stimulus to tones or noise bands to obtain an audiogram.

If the child has a developmental problem such as autism, PDD, or multi-system developmental delay he or she may not respond to speech stimuli. In that case, testing should begin with tones or noise bands. (See Chapter 7, Evaluation of Special Populations.)

Test Order

Test protocol needs to take into consideration the fact that 2-, 3- and 4-year-old children are not always cooperative. Testing should begin with the tasks that require the least amount of cooperation and move on to more difficult tasks as the child becomes more comfortable. It is easiest to begin testing in soundfield because many children initially object to earphones. If a child has anything less than a profound hearing loss she or he should have no problem hearing a stimulus in the soundfield. If testing for conductive hearing loss, begin with a high-frequency stimulus, which should be more easily heard; for sensorineural hearing loss, begin with a low-frequency stimulus because hearing is likely to be better there.

After obtaining at least one low- and one high-frequency threshold, the audiologist must decide what test material is most essential and how likely it is that the child will accept earphones. If testing for conductive hearing loss, and a decision needs to be made about insertion of (PE) tubes, information about separate ear and bone conduction thresholds can be critical. If sensorineural hearing loss is suspected, although separate ear information is valuable, it may be more important to get an idea of the contour of the audiogram before trying earphones. Remember, once you start using earphones, you need to test for twice as many thresholds, and thus to obtain twice as many responses to obtain an audiogram because you must test each frequency in both ears.

When you are ready to try earphone testing, a decision has to be made as to whether to begin with supra-aural earphones or with insert phones. Supra-aural earphones are easy to place on a child quickly. However, they can be heavy for a small head, and even little children are amazingly quick at removing them or pushing them out of their correct position directly over the ear canal. Insert earphones stay in the right place, but they require more effort to insert and poking at the child's ears may be distressing to him or her. The child's acceptance of insert earphones offers the best chance of obtaining good test results.

Regardless of the type of hearing loss suspected, the audiologist should attempt to obtain bone conduction thresholds. Once the child has accepted the bone vibrator, thresholds are usually easy to obtain. If time or attention is a problem, two to three thresholds should be sufficient. When testing for conductive hearing loss, the most critical thresholds are 250, 500, and 2000 Hz. If you reach 2000 Hz and the thresholds no longer indicate conductive hearing loss, additional frequencies should be tested. If the hearing loss is sensorineural, testing at 500, 2000, and 4000 Hz are probably most critical.

Testroom Setup

For many children, testing is most easily accomplished with two testers in a two-room test setup, especially when performing soundfield testing.

However, when earphone testing is to be used, it is frequently easier to have just one tester, who sits next to the child and acts as both tester and test assistant. In this way, the tester has control over the test situation, can interact with the child and facilitate cooperation, and frequently accomplishes testing more quickly. It may be useful to have an audiometer in the test room, which can be used in the following way: At the beginning, while training the child to respond, place the earphones on the test table near him or her and set the signal to a loud level that you are certain the child can hear. Next, train the child to do the task. Once the child is responding reliably, place the earphones on the child's head and proceed in the usual way.

Testing Children with Hearing Loss

Children with mild or moderate hearing losses, or with conductive hearing losses, do not require any special test adaptation except that the audiologist may need to be creative in keeping the child entertained and cooperative during repeat testing. However, children with severe and profound hearing loss may need some test adaptations.

If the child does not respond to soundfield stimuli at the audiometric limits, try testing with a bone vibrator either held in the child's hand or placed on the mastoid. No matter how severe a child's hearing loss is, she or he will feel the vibrator at 250 Hz because this stimulus is tactile, not auditory. Once the child has responded consistently to the tactile stimulus, begin testing with earphones at 250 Hz or 500 Hz; insert earphones are usually preferable if the child will accept them. (For more information, see Chapter 7, Evaluation of Special Populations.)

What To Do if a Child Won't Cooperate

A child is a child. Especially with a very young child, the audiologist should be in control, not the child. If testing cannot be accomplished, the audiologist should accept the responsibility and say, "I was not able to test this child," rather than, "This child is not testable." Having to accept the responsibility for a test failure impels me to try many different approaches before I give up. Although there are some children from whom I cannot get good cooperation, I am willing to try everything I can so that there are very few for whom little or no information is available at the end of a test session.

The answer to the question about what to do if the child won't cooperate starts with what *not* to do. First, do not give up. Take a short rest, have the child go for a walk or a drink at the water fountain, and try again. Try some new toys. Try a new test assistant. Perhaps a parent would be a better test assistant for a particular child. Try using different test stimuli to make the game more interesting. Try a different test room or a different chair. However, do *not* try to use a different test technique. If a child is cognitively at between 3 and 4 years of age, do not try to use VRA. Although the child may initially make a few responses using this technique, he or she will quickly become bored, it will not be possible to obtain more than these few responses, and thus you will not be able to tell if the response was really a threshold response. You can however, use the VRA reinforcers as play reinforcers. Tell the uncooperative child that if she or he cooperates, you will turn on the toy.

Other "bribes," such as stickers, stamps, food, and candy, may also be useful. Promises such as, "After we are finished you can have . . ." work very well. Sometimes, it is useful to offer the treat during testing. If the child seems to be fading, providing occasional reinforcement during the test session (e.g., a piece of a cookie, fruit, raisins, Cheerios, or candy) may prolong the cooperation you receive. If, however, you do not succeed in getting the child to cooperate, it is important that the child not receive the promised reinforcer. If he or she receives the reinforcer after not cooperating, it will make it more difficult to get cooperation in the future.

I believe that parents should participate in all test situations but, for some children, having them in the room reduces cooperation because some parents have a parenting style that does not require children to do things they do not want to do. For some, if the child becomes distressed or frustrated, the parent will remove the child from the situation rather than have the child be distressed. If this is the case, it may be best to have them leave the room and watch from the tester's side. As a last resort, and one that should be used only rarely, I have told children that if they do not cooperate, I will have to send the parents outside. Doing so for a short time may increase the child's cooperation. Although I would not do this on a first visit, it is something that I might consider at a re-evaluation when I cannot complete testing because of the child's uncooperative behavior.

As with all other promises, once you have told a child that you will or will not do something, you must carry it out. If I promise the child a sticker for putting 5 blocks in the box, I should provide the sticker. If I tell the child that he or she cannot leave until the game is over, I need to hold to that. If I tell a child that her or his parents will have to wait outside if she or he does not cooperate, I have to keep my word. In other words, we need to think about what we say to children before we say it, and be prepared to carry out any promises we make.

References and Readings

1. Linden, G., & Harford, E.R. (1985). Keynote address. The pediatric audiologist: From magician to clinician. *Ear Hear, 6,* 6–9.
2. Thompson, M., Thompson G., & Vethivelu, S. (1989). A comparison of audiometric test methods for 2-year-old children. *J Speech Hear Disord, 54,* 174–179.

7

Evaluation of Special Populations

Infants and Children with Severe and Profound Hearing Loss

Children with severe and profound hearing loss who are developing normally should be able to learn auditory test tasks in the same way as their normally hearing peers except that the sound needs to be much louder. It is critical that the audiologist be absolutely certain that the child hears the sound before either turning on the visual reinforcer when using visually reinforced audiometry (VRA), or signaling to the child to respond for play audiometry. Because children with severe and profound hearing loss frequently do not hear sounds, they may not know how to attend to auditory signals. Therefore, it may take more than the usual number of presentations for the child to learn to respond to the conditioning task.

For very young children, testing usually begins in soundfield. If the room is quiet and activities are kept to a minimum, it should be fairly easy to see if the child responds to a loud stimulus. Begin with low-frequency stimuli because hearing-impaired children are likely to hear better at low frequencies. If the child does not respond, try to have the child accept earphones because, in most audiometers, the earphone signal can be about 20 dB louder than the soundfield stimulus. (Centers that see large numbers of children with severe and profound hearing loss may want to consider installing power amplifiers and loudspeakers to permit soundfield testing of louder signals.)

If the child still does not respond, try conditioning the child to a tactile stimulus by placing a bone vibrator in the child's hand or on the mastoid and pairing the tactile and auditory stimuli. Even if the child cannot hear the stimulus, she or he will feel it and become easily conditioned to the task. Once the child is conditioned to the task, try to fade the tactile stimulus. Several attempts may be necessary, but unless the child has no usable hearing, it should be possible to teach the child to respond to an auditory signal using this technique.

Because hearing-impaired children are tested so frequently, they are likely to grow tired of hearing testing, thus the audiologist must be creative to keep the child interested. Changing VRA toys may make them interesting for a little while longer, but this may not have enough of an effect. Placing several reinforcers around the room may keep the child's attention. Using a television (TV) with cartoons as a reinforcer may be more interesting for a two-year-old child. Children with hearing loss frequently learn play audiometry earlier than their normally hearing peers. An interesting and enthusiastic audiologist with several good toys may be able to keep a child's attention long enough to obtain a sufficient number of thresholds using either VRA or play audiometry.

It is not reasonable to expect that any young child will be able to attend long enough to obtain air, bone and speech, acoustic immittance, and hearing aid testing (monaural and binaural) in one test session. Parents need to be told in advance that the audiologist will do as much as possible while the child is cooperating, but that each evaluation will require 2 to 3 test sessions to complete. In my experience, when parents understand that we are trying to maximize the child's functioning, they are understanding about the need for repeat visits.

Infants and Children with Developmental Delay

Unfortunately, having one disability does not prevent a child from having another. Many children with a developmental disability also have a hearing loss. Some of the syndromes and disorders associated with developmental disabilities (e.g., Down syndrome, cytomegalovirus, premature birth) are also associated with impaired hearing. As a result, every child identified with any developmental disability or developmental delay should be followed up audiologically until ear and frequency-specific information has been obtained. If no hearing loss is identified and if the disorder is not a progressive one, the infant can be discharged from follow-up. However, if the disorder has the potential for being progressive (e.g., cytomegalovirus, central nervous system disfunction) or fluctuating (e.g., conductive hearing loss in Down syndrome), the child should be monitored on a regular basis.

It is helpful for the audiologist to learn as much as possible about the specific disorder that the child has because understanding it will help him or her know what disabilities to expect in the child, what types of auditory disorders are likely, and the prognosis for development, speech, and hearing. However, it is important to remember that every disorder presents in variable ways. The developmental delay or the auditory disorder may be mild or severe. Information about the disorder is only a starting place.

As with all children, it is critical to know the cognitive age of an infant or young child to select the appropriate test protocol. Flexer and Gans (1985) demonstrated that by carefully assessing the developmental age of profoundly multihandicapped children, thresholds were obtained at the same levels as those of normally developing children of the same developmental age. This study confirms that developmentally delayed children can be accurately assessed for hearing if developmental age is accurately assessed. When evaluating normally developing children, audiologists make assumptions about developmental age that cannot be made when evaluating children with developmental disabilities. If the child is participating in an educational program, the staff will be able to give the audiologist information about the child's developmental age; the pediatrician may also be able to provide this information. A number of developmental scales are available (see Table 7–1) to assist in making this determination (Katoff, Reuter, & Dunn, 1978; Furuno, O'Reilly, Hosaka, Inastuka, Zeisloft-Falbegy, & Allman, 1978; Furuno, 1984; Blaire, 1975; Pollack, 1997; Brigance, 1991). Once you know the child's cognitive age, you can select the appropriate test protocol: observation, visual reinforcement, or play audiometry.

Positioning

As discussed in the descriptions of specific test protocols, positioning is critical. The infant needs to be positioned so that she or he is comfortable, not straining, and can attend to auditory stimuli. If the child does not have good trunk control, he or she should be seated in a chair that will provide trunk stabilization. Infants can be placed in standard infant seats or leaned against a parent. Older children need adaptive chairs or strollers to provide the support necessary to facilitate head and neck control. Many children are able to turn toward a reinforcement toy if they are seated in a chair that provides stabilization.

A great deal of care needs to be taken in keeping a child with any neurological disorder centered. Normally developing children who have good

Table 7–1.   Tests for Assessing Developmental Level

Brigance, 1991	Brigance Developmental Scale
Furuno et al., 1984	Hawaii Early Learning Profile
Katoff et al., 1978	Kent Infant Development Scale
Blaire, 1975	Language Evaluation Scale
Pollack, 1997	Pollack Developmental Milestones Scale
Frankenburg & Dodds, 1967	The Denver Developmental Screening Test (DDST)

control of their trunk, neck, and head have no difficulty turning more than 90° to look for a reinforcing toy or sitting up to look at the toy if they are bending down. But a child with a neurological disorder and for whom motor activity is difficult will have trouble making a significant head turn. They must be focused facing straight ahead with the visual reinforcer at no more than 90°.

For play audiometry, positioning needs to permit the child optimal range of motion of arms and hands. Some children may need to be held upright to provide upper body support, allowing them use of their arms and hands for the play activity. Play tasks should be carefully selected to be within the child's skill range (e.g., the task of putting pegs into a Peg-Board may be too difficult whereas throwing pegs into a basket may be fine).

Timing of Test Presentation

Delivery of the test signal may require a little more consideration with this population. Because motor control is an issue with many of these children, the audiologist should carefully observe the infant to be certain that he or she is stabilized and comfortable before presenting a stimulus. If the child is squirming and trying to attain a stabilized position, she or he may not be able to respond to a stimulus, and thus, absence of response does not mean inability to hear the stimulus.

Difficulties in Obtaining Responses

Several problems arise in obtaining reliable responses from children with developmental disabilities. The response the child makes may be qualitatively different than a response obtained from normally developing children. For example, it may take a child with a developmental disability longer to focus on a reinforcer and longer to refocus on the distraction toy. There may be a longer latency between presentation of the test stimulus and the response. The audiologist should be sensitive to these differences and change the timing of stimulus presentation accordingly. In some cases, the child may demonstrate a very short latency period, turning almost as soon as the stimulus is presented, which may be an indication of hypersensitivity to sound sensitivity. Motor responses may be slower than with normal children, which also needs to be taken into account. Children with developmental delays may tire more quickly and may habituate to the test stimuli and reinforcers more quickly. They may also fixate on the visual stimulus and it may require a significant effort from the test assistant to center the child's attention after each stimulus presentation. To maximize test results, the test assistant must be aware of the child's mood and change distractors, reinforcers, and play toys quickly to keep the child interested and alert. Social reinforcers are very helpful.

Some children with neurological disorders react negatively to visual reinforcers. When this happens, the audiologist needs to react quickly. Most visual reinforcers allow the audiologist to set the reinforcement toy so that it can be presented with a light only, with light and motion, or with light, motion, and sound. Obviously, if the sound frightens the child, the audiologist should turn off the sound and use only the light or light and motion.

Special Test Procedures

Several test protocols have been developed for use with developmentally delayed children when standard test protocols do not work. One is a tactile–auditory conditioning procedure (Friedlander, Silva, & Knight, 1973; Verpoorten & Emmen, 1995), in which a child is conditioned by pairing a tactile stimulus with an auditory one and the tactile stimulus is gradually withdrawn as the child learns the task. This technique can be performed by using a bone vibrator held in the child's hand or by placing the child's hand on the loudspeaker membrane. The child may remove his or her hand when the stimulus stops, or may make an active response (as in play audiometry) when the stimulus is presented. As the child learns the task, the tactile stimulus fades. Another procedure (Lancioni, Coninx, & Smeets, 1989; Lancioni & Coninx, 1995) uses an air puff paired to an auditory stimulus. The air puff can be directed to the child's face, eyes, or neck and evokes defensive responses such as an eye blink or head turn. An air cylinder is used to supply the air puff.

Infants and Children with Pervasive Developmental Disability

Children with auditory attention disorders, such as those associated with autism, pervasive developmental disorder (PDD), multisystem developmental delay, or regulatory disorders usually have normal hearing but may be unable to attend consistently to auditory stimuli, which is frequently typical of their difficulties in responding to a variety of other sensory stimuli. However, with a little extra effort these children can be reliably tested. For this population, the test setup should be very well controlled. The child needs to be seated in a position in which she or he will not easily be able to walk away. The highchair is ideal. A strong wooden highchair can hold children as old as 7 or 8 years. Although VRA is usually used for children from 5 to 6 to 36 months, this population of children frequently continues to respond to VRA for many years.

Because these children may "tune out" to voices, it is usually best to avoid speech stimuli, at least initially, and to have the test room as quiet as possible. Music, such as the Sesame Street theme or familiar recorded children's songs played through the loudspeaker frequently attracts the child's attention. Once the child has sought out the stimulus, the reinforcer can be activated. The timing of test stimuli is very important with children in this population because they frequently habituate to stimuli quickly. Stimuli should not be presented too close together. This population of children also frequently "tunes out" to auditory stimuli. When a child seems to have "tuned out," it is useful to try different stimuli (noise bands or warble tones), to change the reinforcer toy, or to present very loud stimuli, which may attract the child's attention again and redirect it to the test stimulus. However, some autistic and PDD children are sensitive to loud sounds and presenting one may frighten them. If they are only a little frightened, the loud stimulus may increase their attention, but if they are very upset, it may be difficult to complete testing.

Distraction toys can present a problem for this population. It is important to have the child focused forward but not too involved with the toys. This group of children can be difficult to entertain. If they are more visually than auditorially attentive (which is frequently the case) an interesting toy may cause them to "tune out" to auditory stimuli. Finding the right type of distraction for the individual child requires effort.

Many of these children are sensitive to loud sounds. Their parents report that they have difficulty tolerating sound in the environment and will cry if there is a loud sound, for example, when the family gathers for a party and everyone sings Happy Birthday, or when certain household appliances are turned on. Others will "shut down" if there is too much auditory stimulation, thus it is important that loud stimuli be carefully controlled to keep the child tuned in but not frightened. Stimuli should be presented at low levels and intensity increased gradually. Some children with these disorders ignore sound and almost appear "deaf." For these children, the use of a loud stimulus sometimes helps them "tune in" when their attention has been decreased. Presenting a loud stimulus, sometimes makes the child alert, after which it is possible to get the child to respond to soft stimuli.

Infants and Children with Visual Impairment

Testing visually impaired children with VRA is obviously difficult. If the child cannot see the reinforcer, she or he cannot respond to it. If the child has limited vision, he or she can be moved closer to the reinforcer or the reinforcer can be moved closer to the child to make it easier for the child to see. If this is not sufficient, an alternative is to darken the test room and use a bright flashlight close to the child's face. If the child does not have sufficient vision to see the bright light, a tactile stimulus, such as a vibrator, may be successful. The bone vibrator can be used as the reinforcer by moving the child's hand to the vibrator when the sound is presented. If the child likes the vibrator, she or he will make the association and reach for it at the sound. The air puff technique described earlier for children with developmental delays may be useful. Blind children functioning at the 3-year-old level or above should be able to perform play audiometry tasks by selecting toys that do not require difficult manipulation.

Graduates of the Neonatal Intensive Care Nursery

Neonatal Intensive Care Unit (NICU) graduates need to be evaluated in the same way other infants are. Research by Smith, Zimmerman, Connolly, Jerger, & Yelich (1992) indicated that as many as 35% of NICU graduates may have hearing loss, which makes it clear that hearing testing of this population is critical. Testing should be delayed until the infant is stable, and is frequently delayed until a few days before hospital discharge. However, if the infant is to be hospitalized for several months, it is necessary to test him or her earlier than discharge so that if there is hearing impairment, the infant will not be functioning without auditory stimulation during critical developmental months. It is very important that every attempt be made to identify if hearing loss is present and to fit the infant with appropriate amplification.

Although NICU graduates are evaluated in the same way as other infants, there may be additional testing difficulties. As with other infants, it is critical to obtain an accurate developmental age and use the appropriate test protocol. Some NICU graduates function like children with developmental delays and will need the same considerations as those suggested for that population. Many have feeding problems and may not suck. If that is the case, it will be very difficult to do observation audiometry, but air puff audiometry may be possible (see earlier section on developmental delay). NICU babies live in a very noisy environment and, as a result, may not attend to sound. The audiologist who works with NICU patients may be able to assist in monitoring the auditory environment and in helping to control noise levels.

Children with Functional Hearing Loss

It is not unusual for children between the ages of 8 and 12 years to occasionally demonstrate functional hearing losses. Typically, a child fails a hearing screening either in school or in the pediatrician's office and is referred to an audiologist for a complete evaluation. The audiologist may suspect that the hearing loss is functional if the following are present: (a) speech reception thresholds are much better or worse than pure-tone thresholds; (b) responses to speech stimuli are unusual (e.g., consistently saying only half of the spondee); (c) test results do not agree with the child's ability to communicate (i.e., the child seems to understand with no difficulty although thresholds indicate a moderately severe hearing loss, or she or he has a great deal of difficulty communicating when thresholds are near normal); (d) test results are not repeatable; or (e) unmasked bone conduction thresholds are much poorer in one ear than in the other.

If you suspect a functional hearing loss, try first to reinstruct the child. Tell the child, "Maybe you did not understand the directions. This is hard to do. You need to raise your hand even if the sound is very, very soft." Alternatively, you can suggest that there may be something wrong with the equipment, which is causing the problem. "There must be something wrong with this equipment. It is making it seem that you have much worse hearing than I know you have. Let's go into a different test room and try again." You are not exactly telling the child that you think he or she is faking the hearing loss but you are making it clear that the results are not accurate.

If you do not get test results reflecting cooperation on the second try, you may have to rely on alternative techniques to get results. It is very useful to use a portable audiometer and have the child seated next to you so that you can make eye contact. It is much more difficult for a child to say that she or he does not hear a sound when looking you in the eye.

If the child's responses still are not providing accurate results, have the child "count the beeps." Tell the child that he or she will hear 1, 2, or 3 beeps and to tell you how many she or he hears. Start at a level that the child admits to hearing. For example, if the child admits to hearing at 40 dB, present 2 beeps at 40 dB and when the child says, "Two," present 2 beeps at 40 dB and 1 beep at 35 dB. If the child responds, "Three," you know that the child heard 3 beeps and heard at both 35 dB and 40 dB. Continue in this fashion until you obtain consistent responses.

Obtaining the audiogram is actually the easy part. Now you must explain the test results to both child and parent. You could simply say that the child has normal hearing and send him or her home, but that may be begging the issue. Why did the child feel the need to simulate a hearing loss?

Once you have taken this "crutch" away, will the child substitute something else? It is probably useful to tell the child that she or he has normal hearing. However, it is important to discuss with the parents or caregiver that the child may be having difficulties that are causing stress and suggest that they find out if anything is bothering the child. It is possible that simply being aware that the child is under stress will help them provide the necessary support. If not, telling them the results can alert them to seek help.

Conclusion

Children with all types of developmental, behavior, and auditory disorders are testable. A review of the literature and the experiences of many pediatric audiologists clearly indicate that test results can be obtained on almost any child. The audiologist has to believe that she or he can test the child and be creative in finding ways to accomplish the task. The reward of accurately assessing the hearing of a child who is difficult to evaluate is well worth the effort.

References and Readings

Berk, R.L., & Feldman, A.S. (1958). Functional hearing loss in children. *New Engl J Med, 259,* 214–216.

Blaire, F.X. (1975). *Language Evaluation Scale.* Milwaukee, WI: Department of Special Education, University of Wisconsin, Milwaukee.

Brigance, A. (1991). *Diagnostic Inventory of Early Development Curriculum.* North Billerica, MA: Associates Incorporated.

Flexer, C., & Gans, D.P. (1985). Comparative evaluation of the auditory responsiveness of normal infants and profoundly multihandicapped children. *J Speech Hear Res, 28,* 163–168.

Frankenburg, W., & Dodds, J. (1967). The Denver Developmental Screening Test. *J Pediatr, 71,* 181.

Friedlander, B.Z., Silva, D.A., & Knight, M.S. (1973). Selective responses to auditory and auditory-vibratory stimuli by severely retarded deaf-blind children. *J Aud Res, 13,* 105–111.

Furuno, S., O'Reilly, K.A., Hosaka, C.M., Inastuka, T.T., Zeisloft-Falbegy, B., & Allman, T. (1984). *Hawaii Early Profile (Help Check List).* Palo Alto, CA: Vort Corporation.

Hayes, D., & Northern, J.L. (1996). *Infants and Hearing.* San Diego: Singular Publishing.

Katoff, L., Reuter, J., & Dunn, V. (1978). *The Kent Infant Developmental Scale Manual.* Kent, OH: Kent State University.

Kile, J.E. (1996). Audiologic assessment of children with Down syndrome. *Am J Audiol, 5,* 44–52.

Lancioni, G.E., Coninx, F., & Smeets, P.M. (1989). A classical conditioning procedure for the hearing assessment of multihandicapped persons. *J Speech Hear Res, 54,* 88–93.

Lancioni, G.E., & Coninx, F. (1995). A classical condition procedure for auditory testing: air puff audiometry. *Scand Audiol, 24,* (Suppl. 41), 43–48.

Northern, J.L., & Downs, M. (1991). *Hearing in Children* (4th ed.). Baltimore: Williams & Wilkins.

Pollack, J. (1997). *Developmental Milestones Scale.* Brooklyn, NY: Lamm Institute, Long Island College Hospital.

Smith, R.J.H., Zimmerman, B., Connolly, P.K., Jerger, S.W., & Yelich, A. (1992). Screening audiometry using the high-risk register in a level III nursery. *Arch Otolaryngol Head Neck Surg, 118,* 1306–1311.

Verpoorten, R.A., & Emmen, J.G. (1995). A tactile-auditory conditioning procedure for the hearing assessment of persons with autism and mental retardation. *Scand Audiol, 24,* (Suppl. 41), 49–50.

8

The Role of the Test Assistant

When evaluating infants and young children, testing is frequently more easily accomplished with two examiners. Both examiners may be audiologists, or one may be an audiologists and one a test assistant. If they are both audiologists, they can alternate roles, taking turns behind the audiometer and interacting with the child.

However, whether one or two testers is involved in any test situation, only one audiologist is in charge. The managing audiologist (for want of a better term), usually the person sitting in front of the audiometer, must determine test protocol, presentation mode, order of testing, and timing of presentations. Occasionally, the person working with the child may be the managing audiologist and give directions to the test assistant, who is sitting behind the audiometer and presenting test stimuli. This may occur with a difficult-to-test child when test order and timing may make a difference in whether or not testing is accomplished and when the managing audiologist has had more experience with difficult children.

Working with Parents

The test assistant is responsible for engaging the infant or child, keeping the child interested and attentive, and keeping family members at ease so they can cooperate with test protocols. The test assistant should first be certain that family members understand what is being tested, how testing is accomplished, and what their role will be. The child may be seated on a parent's lap or in an infant seat, highchair, or in a chair at a test table. The parent may be seated next to the child or slightly behind him or her to be able to observe, but not distract, the child. If the child is uncomfortable with strangers, the parent may be the best person to play with the child, with some direction from the test assistant.

The first responsibility of the test assistant is to explain the test protocol to the family. Describe what will be done (observation, visual reinforcement, play, standard), what will be expected of the child, and what will be expected of them. Family members need to understand that they must appear interested but not respond to any test stimuli before the child responds so that the audiologist can be certain of measuring the child's hearing, not his or her ability to receive cues from parents. It is frequently difficult for parents to sit still and not react when the child does not seem to be responding to the presentation of test stimuli. They may have to be instructed not to say, "Did you hear that?" or to look expectantly at the child when sounds are presented. When speech stimuli are used, the parents may need be reminded that they cannot repeat the tester's stimuli for the child (e.g., "She said, 'baseball', say, 'baseball' ") when the child fails to respond. If the child is looking to them or the test assistant for encouragement, it may be best to look away from the child, and at the toy, the loudspeaker, or the floor so the child understands that they will not provide cues about when to respond. Once family members understand that their behavior may make it difficult to obtain reliable results, they are usually willing to do whatever is needed. The use of noise-canceling earphones may be effective in reducing extraneous responses from family members.

Observation Audiometry

For observation audiometry, both the managing audiologist and the test assistant must have a good view of the infant so that both can judge if a response is present. If the infant is in an infant seat, either the test assistant or other adult may be holding the bottle. If the infant is being nursed or is not comfortable in an infant seat, she or he can be in the mother's arms. If the parent is holding the infant or the bottle, the test assistant needs to be certain that there is no change in the way the bottle or the breast is held, or that it is moving in or out of the infant's mouth when sound stimuli are presented. The test assistant needs to be certain that the infant is seated comfortably and not fidgeting. If may be helpful for him or her to hold and to manipulate a bright toy in front of the infant to keep the infant focused straight ahead and to reduce fidgeting.

When a sound is presented, both the test assistant and managing audiologist need to judge the presence of a response. The test assistant should be careful about how she or he informs the managing audiologist about the observation. The testers need to work out a discreet signal system such as a slight head nod indicating yes or no, or finger movement (1 finger for yes, 2 for no). If the test assistant repeatedly says, "No, I didn't see anything," it is likely to be disturbing to the family. Because the test assistant is right next to the infant he or she will be able to make suggestions about when a rest or a repositioning may be needed.

Visual Reinforcement Audiometry

In visual reinforcement audiometry (VRA) the test assistant's responsibility is to assist in training the child to the task and then keep the child focused straight ahead so the child can make a conditioned head turn. Positioning is especially important for young children and for children with neurological and developmental delays. The test assistant should be certain that the child is comfortably seated, has sufficient neck support, and is facing forward. If the child is turned to one side and sound stimuli are being presented and reinforced from the other side, it may be difficult to get good responses. Focusing the child forward is most easily accomplished if the test assistant is seated in front of the child, but in a position that permits the managing audiologist also to see the child. The distraction toys the test assistant selects should be easily manipulable, bright, entertaining, and quiet. As soon as the child starts to lose interest and look away, a new toy should be presented.

When training the child for the VRA task, the tester keeps the child's attention focused to the front and attracts the child to the reinforcing toy when it is turned on. Once the child has been trained, the test assistant keeps the child focused forward and away from the reinforcing toy. The child should be observing and not manipulating the toy because this may be too engrossing, especially for young children. As children get older they may be able to play with simple toys and still respond to sound. The test assistant needs to be alert and aware of whether playing with toys is interfering with the child's attention. If it is, the tester should take the toys away from the child.

The test room does not have to be silent during testing but it should be quiet. Speech should be at a minimum. The amount of interaction the tester and child have will depend partly on the personality of the tester and partly on that of the child. For some children, smiling, clapping and enthusiastic comments of "Hurrah!" will encourage longer attention to the VRA task. For other children, these will be an interference and better results will be obtained if the test assistant is quiet or even silent. A silent test assistant is frequently preferable with a child with pervasive developmental disorder (PDD) or other developmental disorders. The test assistant needs to observe the child and determine what mode of behavior produces the best results.

Play Audiometry

With play audiometry, the test assistant teaches the child the task and assists the child in completing the test activities. The test assistant must judge the child's motor skills and select toys that she or he is capable of using, note when the child's interest is flagging, and determine when a new toy is needed. For children who do not wish to cooperate, the test assistant needs to present a firm, but kind, attitude to increase cooperation, and must determine when to involve parents in getting cooperation and when it is best to leave the parents out. As with VRA, the amount of interaction the tester and child have will depend partly on the personality of the tester and partly on that of the child. However, because children who do play are older, more interaction is to be expected.

Speech Audiometry

The use of a test assistant can be critical for speech audiometry. If a closed-set task is being used, the test assistant will be responsible for turning pages and being certain that the managing audiologist knows how the child responded. If an open-set format is being used and the child is repeating the test stimulus, the test assistant may need to be the audiologist's "ears," especially if the child is responding in the very soft voice typical of many young children. The test assistant needs to find a way to let the audiologist know if the response was correct or not, and if the audiologist is doing phoneme scoring, to tell the audiologist what the error was without making the child feel as if he or she is doing poorly at the task. There are several ways to accomplish this. The test assistant can simply repeat what the child said in a voice sufficiently loud for the audiologist to hear, or repeat just the error words. For example, if the stimulus item is, "You will say mouth," and the child says, "mouse," the test assistant repeats, "mouse." The audiologist will know that an error was made, will be able to record what the error was, and the child will not feel that she or he is failing at the task.

Keeping Order in the Test Room

An important responsibility for the test assistant is keeping the test room in order. When a child is brought into a test room, most of the toys should be out of sight. One or two toys should be there to entice the child to enter and to sit in the test chair. If you bring a young child, especially a difficult-to-evaluate child, into a room that has toys all over the floor, it will be difficult to get the child seated, and it is difficult to get the child's attention focused on what you are doing. When toys are put away, they should be sorted appropriately, being certain that all parts are in the correct boxes. Using a Peg-Board or a puzzle with a missing piece may result in annoyance or frustration for the child, as can having toy cars mixed up with Lego pieces. These situations end up wasting time while the child discusses what is missing and why things are in the wrong place or while she or he simply examines each piece before using it to determine what it is. For some children, this will be so distressing that it may interfere with testing.

Conclusion

The test assistant is critical to obtaining good results. An enthusiastic, cheerful test assistant who enjoys children is more likely to get good results. When the test assistant and the managing audiologist disagree or are not communicating well, it is probably best if they take a moment to leave the test room and discuss how they want to proceed, out of earshot of the family. It hardly encourages confidence if the testers cannot agree about what to do. An experienced team makes the task easier to accomplish.

9

Speech Audiometry*

Purpose of Speech Audiometry

Speech audiometry, appropriately used, can be an extremely valuable part of the clinical audiological test battery, particularly for evaluating and monitoring auditory function in children. Pure-tone testing provides information about degree and type of hearing loss, but does not provide information about function—how a person is able to use hearing for perception of speech, which is critical for the development of language and accurate speech production. Speech perception testing is the only method available for assessing how a child understands speech. Unfortunately, it is frequently overlooked or used in a limited fashion, thereby failing to maximize its potential usefulness.

Assessing speech perception can be very helpful in determining what kind of difficulties a child has, and in planning remediation. Word-recognition scores that are poorer than expected when compared to pure-tone thresholds at normal and soft conversational levels can be strong indicators for aggressive treatment: medical or audiological. Testing at soft conversational levels and in the presence of competing noise can effectively demonstrate the need for hearing aids, for a frequency modulation (FM) system in the classroom, or for auditory training. Information available from evaluation of large numbers of adults indicates that word-recognition ability decreases as the degree of hearing loss increases. This is also true for children (Boothroyd, 1984). However, the effect of hearing loss is much more significant for children than for adults because of the negative impact that even a mild hearing loss can have on the development of speech and language

*This chapter is adapted with permission from Madell, J.R. (1995). Speech audiometry for children. In: Gerber, S.E. (ed.). *The Handbook of Pediatric Audiology* (pp 84–103). Washington, D.C.: Gallaudet University Press.

(Ross & Giolas, 1978; Wallace, Gravel, McCarton, & Ruben, 1988; Friel-Patti, Finito-Hieber, Conti, & Brown, 1982, Clopton & Silverman, 1977). Word-recognition testing evaluates the extent to which a child's hearing loss has adversely affected her or his speech perception, putting development of speech and language at risk.

For children who have been identified with hearing losses or auditory processing disorders, word-recognition testing is useful in monitoring progress during treatment. Almost everyone agrees that, regardless of the mode of communication in which families choose to educate their hearing-impaired children, all children should be given the opportunity to maximize their auditory skills. Providing appropriate amplification is a necessary, but incomplete, step toward this goal. Children must be taught to use residual hearing for perception of speech. Even young children with profound hearing losses can be taught to use audition for the reception of language. The use of audition will positively affect language growth and improve speech production. The audiologist who evaluates a child annually, semiannually, or quarterly may be in a better position to evaluate auditory progress than the therapist or teacher who sees the child several times a week. If a therapy program is successful, the child's word recognition should continue to improve and, over time, the child should be able to perform more difficult auditory tasks. During routine evaluations, the audiologist can monitor the child's progress and assist the therapist in modifying treatment goals to improve the child's auditory functioning. This, to my mind, is one of the most exciting areas of pediatric audiology.

Evaluating Auditory Perception

The goal of speech audiometry is to obtain as much information as possible about a child's speech perception abilities. There are several ways to evaluate speech perception, and each procedure provides different information. Erber (1976, 1979) describes an auditory skills matrix that is useful when thinking about the different components of speech-perception testing and auditory listening tasks.

There are four different response tasks that can be used to assess perception. *Detection* is the ability to tell when a stimulus is present. *Discrimination* is the ability to determine if two stimuli are the same or different. *Identification* is the ability to recognize the stimulus being presented and to identify it by repeating, pointing, or writing. *Comprehension* is the ability to understand what the stimulus means.

Each response task can be assessed using a number of different stimuli, from phonemes, syllables, words, phrases, and sentences, to connected discourse. Phoneme testing is the most difficult task in the stimulus hierarchy because it is less redundant and provides the fewest cues; however, it provides valuable information. Phoneme testing can be presented in either a closed- or open-set format and provides specific information about which sounds are incorrectly perceived; also, many stimuli can be tested in a short period of time. Connected discourse, on the other hand, is easier to understand, but will provide very little information about which specific phonemes are causing perceptual difficulties because the listener may correctly extrapolate words she or he does not correctly perceive from contextual cues.

Erber (1979) suggests that to assess fully a person's speech-perception abilities, it is necessary to utilize all the different stimuli, using each response task. The resulting complex evaluation will provide the kind of complete information that is necessary to fully understand each child's auditory functioning and is invaluable in planning an auditory training program for a child with impaired hearing or an auditory processing disorder. Fortunately, because of the time it requires, it is not a necessary part of every audiological evaluation. However, it is useful for the audiologist to keep the auditory skills matrix in mind when selecting tests for evaluating a particular child and for determining which tests and how many tests are needed to assess fully each child's auditory functioning.

Factors to Consider when Selecting Speech-Perception Tests

Closed Set versus Open-Set Testing

Word-recognition tests may be divided into two categories: closed-set tests and open-set tests. In closed-set testing, the number of possible items is restricted. The child being tested understands what all the possible test stimuli are and will select her or his response from that limited number of potential items. Items might be numbers, body parts, alphabet letters, or pictures placed in front of the child. Open-set testing provides no clues. The child may know that the stimulus will be a 1-, 2-, or 3-syllable word,

Table 9–1.   Factors To Consider in Selecting Speech Audiometry Tests

Closed set vs open set
Vocabulary level
Degree of hearing loss
Phoneme scoring vs whole-word scoring
Half vs full lists
Use of a carrier phrase
Recorded vs monitored, live-voice testing
Number of tests needed
Use of visual cues

but will know nothing else about it. Any word in his or her vocabulary is a possibility. In some cases, the child may be asked to repeat what she or he hears, even if it isn't a word. Open-set testing is much more difficult than closed-set testing, and frequently results in lower scores, but may provide a more realistic picture of speech-perception abilities in conversation.

Vocabulary Level

It is essential that the tester know the child's vocabulary level to select the appropriate test. If possible, determine the child's vocabulary age by using a standardized vocabulary test, by obtaining information from tests done at another evaluation, or from reporting by parents, caregivers, or teachers. When the above alternatives are not available, use information obtained from observation and conversation with the child. Selecting test materials that contain vocabulary that is not in the child's lexicon will result in a score that is not a true reflection of her or his speech perception abilities. It may be helpful to ask parents to tell you if you use a word they think the child does not know so that you can substitute another word. Occasionally, the child does know the word (from school or from therapists) and the parents are not aware of it.

Degree of Hearing Loss

Degree of hearing loss should not be a factor in selecting tests of speech perception. Tests should be selected based on the individual child's abilities. It is unfair to the child to make assumptions about how he or she will be able to perform based on the pure-tone audiogram alone. Many children with profound hearing losses are capable of using residual hearing for reception of auditory information. However, it is undoubtedly true that profound hearing loss makes it more difficult to receive information using the auditory channel. For children who have not had the opportunity for early intervention, who have not been trained in a program that emphasizes the use of audition, or who do not have the ability to use audition, special tests have been developed that make word recognition testing possible (see section on Word-Recognition Tests for Severe and Profound Hearing Loss later in this chapter).

Phoneme Scoring versus Whole-Word Scoring

Most of the tests that we use to evaluate speech perception are scored according to whether or not the person has correctly identified the whole word. If the person makes an error on one phoneme, the entire word is scored as wrong. This method of scoring may be depriving us of useful information. Arthur Boothroyd (1968, 1984, 1988) has written extensively about phoneme scoring and its advantages and has developed tests that rely on phoneme scoring. But phoneme scoring can be used with any test. By recording the phoneme errors that a child makes during any speech-perception test, we can learn what parts of the spectrum are not being appropriately perceived. Vowel errors indicate insufficient low-frequency information, inability to perceive sibilants correctly indicates insufficient high-frequency information, or possible upward spread of masking caused by too much low-frequency amplification. Knowing the specific spectral bands of the sibilants that are misperceived will provide even more specific information. Such information may permit us to make changes in the frequency response of the child's amplification system, to make earmold modifications, and to make suggestions about auditory training goals.

Half-list versus Full List

The issue of half list versus full list has been debated in the field of audiology for some time. Obviously, using a full 50-word list reduces the chance of error in scoring. However, when working with young children, a number of factors need to be considered. With young children, time is of the essence. It is necessary to obtain a great deal of information in a short period of time, and it may not be possible to obtain all the necessary test results if too much time is spent on any one test. However, the necessity for speed does not permit using less than the required number of stimuli to obtain reliable results. Short lists should only be used when that protocol has been validated. The number of words used must be sufficient to obtain all the information necessary to assess the child's speech-perception abilities. This assessment can usually be achieved with 25 words on most tests but not with 10. Except in rare cases like the Isophonemic Word Lists (Boothroyd, 1968) which have been standardized as 10 word- (30-phoneme) lists, 10 words will not provide a sufficient number or variety of stimuli to obtain an accurate score.

Use of a Carrier Phrase

Most word-recognition tasks were designed to be used with a carrier phrase. The carrier phrase alerts the child to attend and places the word in a sentence context that more accurately represents its use in normal conversation. The carrier phrase usually ends with a vowel so that the carrier phrase does not influence the word. Common carrier phrases are "you will say," "show me the," or "tell me."

Recorded versus Monitored Live Voice

Recorded testing has the advantage of being more easily comparable from test session to test session. It also avoids the possibility of the tester modifying her or his voice either intentionally or unintentionally to assist the child in obtaining a higher score. On the other hand, recorded testing is more time consuming, and prevents the audiologist from making adaptions that are sometimes needed when testing children. Children may need more "off time" between stimuli to be able to attend than the recording permits, may need to have an item repeated if they get distracted and begin to talk to a parent or the tester, and may need time out for encouragement. It is certainly possible to stop a tape or compact disc (CD) player and rewind, but this is often difficult to accomplish efficiently. My experience has indicated that if the tester is aware of the pitfalls of live-voice testing, it is possible to obtain accurate results using monitored, live voice.

Is One Test Enough?

With both children and adults, optimal information will be obtained by using more than one test during an evaluation. Figure 9–1 contains test results of a child with a profound hearing loss. Word-recognition testing with a 4-item forced choice, closed-set test (Northwestern University Children's Hearing in Pictures [NU-CHIPS]) indicated that he had excellent word-recognition skills with his FM system. Because this is a closed-set test, the results may not be a realistic assessment of how he will do in conversation. A repeat test in an open-set format (no pictures) indicated that he had much poorer skills than the closed-set test had indicated. Both tests provided important information and taken together, give an accurate picture of this child's auditory skills. Figure 9–2 contains the test results for a child who appeared to have very poor word-recognition abilities when using open-set testing. When closed-set testing was performed, it became clear that he had some word-recognition abilities. The additional use of phoneme scoring can provide even more useful information, telling us which sounds the child can perceive correctly and which he or she cannot. Based on this information, we can modify amplification to provide more emphasis in the frequency areas where perception is poor and can stress these phonemes in auditory training.

Using Visual Clues

Most speech perception testing is performed using audition alone. However, when a child has very poor word-recognition skills or has very little confidence in her or his auditory abilities, it may be useful to test using vision alone, audition alone, and both vision and audition together. When testing using vision and audition, the child is permitted to watch the face of the examiner and listen at the same time, permitting a combined approach to listening that is more similar to what is experienced in daily activities. However, it is important to obtain information using audition alone because only that information will provide the necessary information for setting am-

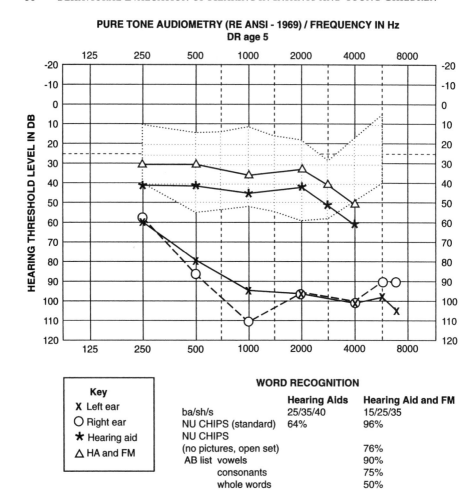

Figure 9–1. Word-recognition testing comparing open- and closed-set testing and phoneme scoring for a child with a profound hearing loss.

plification and for planning auditory training. By testing using vision alone and comparing the scores to the combined vision–audition test, it is possible to know how much each sense contributes to reception of speech.

Threshold Speech Tests

Audiologists frequently begin evaluations with adults using pure-tone stimuli, but many pediatric audiologists begin with speech stimuli. Any

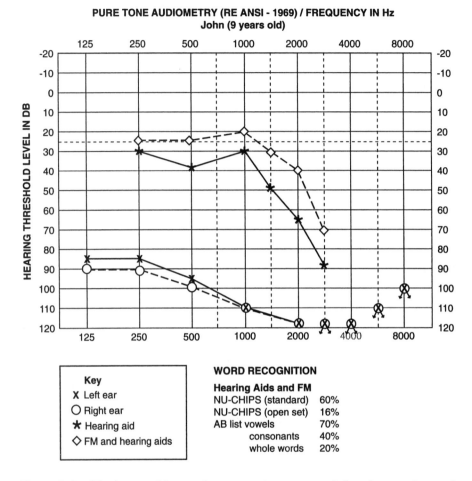

Figure 9–2. Word-recognition testing comparing open- and closed-set testing, and phoneme scoring for a child with a profound hearing loss.

audiologist who works with children is aware that speech, probably because of its familiarity and interest, can more easily attract the attention of a young child than can pure-tone or noise-band stimuli. The stimulus used will be determined by the child's speech and language skills. Speech-awareness thresholds or speech-recognition thresholds provide basic information about auditory status, and can be useful in determining at what level to begin when presenting pure-tone or noise-band stimuli for threshold testing, and to confirm pure-tone thresholds.

Table 9–2.   Speech-Threshold Tests

Speech-Awareness/Detection Tests
   Conversational voice
   Music
   5-sound test *(a,i,u,sh,s)*; Ling, 1978
   3-sound test *(ba,sh,s)*; Madell, 1990
Speech Reception Threshold Tests
   Body parts
   Familiar toys or objects
   Numbers
   Spondee pictures
   Spondee words (standard protocol)
   Threshold by Identification of Pictures (TIP);
      Siegenthaler & Haspiel, 1966

Speech-Awareness or Speech-Detection Thresholds

The speech-awareness threshold (SAT) or speech-detection threshold (SDT) is a test that uses speech stimuli to determine threshold—the softest level at which a person can detect the presence of the stimulus 50% of the time. SATs are usually used only when more complex speech stimuli cannot be used, such as when testing a very young child who does not have the vocabulary for other speech testing, or when testing a person with extremely poor or no word-recognition ability.

A variety of different stimuli can be used. The most common stimulus is conversational voice. The audiologist may call the child's name or use music either by singing or using recorded children's songs. However, the information obtained will be limited, since both music and conversation are broad-band stimuli. The threshold obtained will be close to the threshold at the frequency that the child hears the softest. More useful information is obtained by using the Ling Five-Sound Test (Ling, 1978). The test items are selected to provide frequency specific information and include *a, i, u, sh,* and *s*. The vowels assess perception of low-frequency stimuli, *sh* assesses perception of mid-high frequency stimuli, and *s* assesses perception of high-frequency stimuli. An adapted version (Madell, 1990) uses *ba* or *bu* for assessing low-frequency stimuli, *sh* for assessing mid–high-frequency stimuli, and *s* for assessing high-frequency stimuli. Although it takes slightly longer to obtain these three thresholds than it does to obtain one, the information obtained is much more valuable than that obtained using a single, broad-frequency stimulus. It is frequency specific and provides information about how a person can be expected to perceive speech stimuli across the frequency range needed for speech. In addition, because the test is frequency specific, it can be more directly compared to pure-tone thresholds.

Speech-Recognition Thresholds

The speech recognition threshold (SRT) determines the softest level at which a person can identify speech stimuli 50% of the time. It differs from detection tasks, which only require that the person be aware of the presence of speech, not identify it. The test materials selected will depend on the individual being tested. When possible, it is desirable to use test materials and procedures that are standardized on adults so that results are comparable. This will obviously not be possible with all children, but the fact that it is not possible does not mean that you cannot obtain useful information. Older children with good language skills will be able to perform well on the standard tests that were developed for adults. Young children may not have the vocabulary or may be too shy to repeat back what the tester has said. For these children, a picture-pointing task or a task requiring pointing to body parts will be easier and will produce useful results.

The test procedure for SRTs requires that the person be familiar with the material being presented. Familiarity will make testing easier and result in a threshold at a softer level than that obtained with open-set testing in which any vocabulary word might be used. Standard testing uses spondee words (two-syllable words with equal stress on both syllables.) With children who can perform this task, the audiologist reads the list of words at a comfortably loud level, permitting speechreading if necessary, with the child repeating the word to verify that the word has been understood. Once the child is familiar with the words, the audiologist begins testing using audition alone, and reduces the intensity until the child begins making errors. The audiologist then ascends and descends, establishing the level at which the child can correctly repeat the words 50% of the time. American Speech-Language-Hearing Association (ASHA) guidelines for speech–recognition-threshold testing (1988) describe a complex procedure that, while resulting in an accurate threshold, may be too time consuming for use with some children. Cramer and Erber (1974) found that the best results were obtained by asking the child to say the word and point at the same time. This combined task may increase the child's attention to the task and result in improved scores.

For children who cannot perform using standard techniques, the audiologist can use pictures or objects of the spondee words. The presence of the items will make the task easier. If the child's vocabulary is not sufficient for the use of standard spondees, similar information can be obtained using familiar objects, pictures, or body parts. Even very young children less than 2 years of age are likely to be able to point to eyes, nose, mouth, ears, hair, and shoes, for example. For children whose speech perception is very poor, it may be possible to obtain an SRT using numbers from 1 to 10 because number recognition requires only vowel perception.

Siegenthaler and Haspiel (1966) developed a threshold test, Threshold by the Identification of Pictures (TIP). It is a picture-identification test that uses monosyllabic words rather than the standard bisyllabic words. Monosyllabic words are less redundant than bisyllabic words, which makes the task more difficult and may affect test results adversely.

Word-Recognition Testing

These tests are designed to evaluate a child's ability to understand speech under different listening conditions. Unlike threshold testing, word-recognition testing is performed at suprathreshold levels. Testing may be conducted at different intensities and under varying conditions of competing noise. The selection of test materials and test conditions will depend on the child's vocabulary level and the child's ability to cooperate. Scoring requires accurate perception of all the phonemes in any word to obtain a correct score. By modifying the response task and types of reinforcement, it is possible to learn a great deal about a child's speech-perception skills. No audiological evaluation is complete without obtaining some speech-perception information.

Closed-Set Word-Recognition Tests

NUMBERS

Identification of numbers may be the easiest word-recognition task because the vocabulary is familiar to most children and only requires vowel recognition. Erber (1980) developed a test, the ANT (Auditory Numbers Test), that used pictures of 1, 2, 3, 4, or 5 ants on cards with corresponding numbers from 1 to 5. This is simply a more formalized way of testing number recognition, but the pictures may hold more interest for young children than does simply repeating numbers.

BODY PARTS OR OTHER FAMILIAR OBJECTS

Pointing to body parts is an easy task even for very young children, and can usually be made into an interesting game. The child can point to his or her body parts, to a doll's, or to a parent's. This same task can also be accomplished using pictures or objects with which the child is familiar. Because only a limited number of stimuli is being used, the results must be interpreted with care.

AUDITORY PERCEPTION OF ALPHABET LETTERS

The Auditory Perception of Alphabet Letters (APAL) test was developed to overcome the difficulties caused by reduced vocabulary in many children with impaired hearing and to evaluate the type of errors the child is mak-

Table 9–3. Word-Recognition Tests

Closed-Set Tests
Numbers
Auditory Numbers Test (ANT); Erker, 1980
Body parts/familiar objects
Alphabet Test (APAL); Ross & Randolph, 1990
Northwestern University Children's Hearing Pictures (NU-CHIPS); Elliot &   Katz, 1980
Word Intelligibility by Picture Identification (WIPI); Ross & Lerman, 1997
Discrimination in Pictures (DIP); Siegenthaler & Haspiel, 1966
Pediatric Speech Intelligibility Test (PSI); Jerger & Jerger, 1982
Speech Patterns Contrast Test (SPAC); Boothroyd, 1984, 1987
Open-Set Tests
NU-CHIPS words without pictures
WIPI words without pictures
Phonetically Balanced Kindergarten List (PBK); Haskins, 1949
Isophonemic word lists (AB Lists); Boothroyd, 1968
Connected discourse testing

ing (Ross & Randolph, 1990) and requires that the child be able to identify spoken letters of the alphabet. Responses may be made orally, using finger spelling, or by pointing to a response board. A recorded version of the test is available. The tester uses the carrier phrase, "The letters are," and then says 2 letters. The child must identify the 2 letters in sequence. The scoring sheet provides 3 weighted categories, developed to analyze errors in terms of their perceptual distance from the stimulus. For example, if the stimulus is p and the child identifies t he or she is off by only one distinctive feature (voicing) and this is a Category I error. If the response is off by 2 features (e.g., voicing and place or manner) it is a Category II error, and all other errors are Category III errors. The test form permits easy scoring. Children who make primarily Category I errors have relatively good perception that could benefit from training. Children with Category II or III errors are having more difficulty with auditory perception and will require more training.

NORTHWESTERN UNIVERSITY CHILDREN'S HEARING IN PICTURES

The NU-CHIPS, developed by Elliot and Katz, (1980), is a 4-item, forced-choice picture-identification test. It has 50 stimulus pages and can be used in whole-list or half-list format. Two versions are available, providing a total of four 50-word lists or eight 25-word lists. The vocabulary is at the 3-year-old level and can frequently be used with two-year-olds. A recorded version is available with a choice of either a man or a woman speaking.

WORD INTELLIGIBILITY BY PICTURE IDENTIFICATION

The Word Intelligibility by Picture Identification (WIPI), developed by Ross and Lerman (1970), is a 6-item, forced-choice picture-identification test with 25 items and 4 test forms. This test requires the vocabulary of a three-and-a-half-year-old and is available in recorded format. It is slightly more difficult than the NU-CHIPS because it is a 6-item test and the vocabulary is more difficult. It is a good alternative for slightly older children. Some of the pictures on both tests are difficult to recognize. The picture of the church in the WIPI is difficult to identify. The word "purse" in the NU-CHIPS is not one used in the northeastern United States.

DISCRIMINATION IN PICTURES

The Discrimination in Pictures (DIP), developed by Siegenthaler and Haspiel (1966) is a 2-item, forced-choice picture identification test containing 48 pairs of monosyllabic words. Because there are only 2 choices for each item, there is a 50% chance of randomly answering the item correctly, which makes interpreting the test results difficult.

PEDIATRIC SPEECH INTELLIGIBILITY TEST

The Pediatric Speech Intelligibility ([PSI] Jerger & Jerger, 1982) is a picture-pointing test designed to provide both central and peripheral auditory processing information and intended to assist in locating sites of lesion. The test uses both monosyllabic words and sentence materials and tests performance-intensity functions and message-to-competition functions. Sentences form the competing message. The test comes in a 5-tape version and a 3-tape screening version and is intended to be used in a recorded format only. The test is designed to be used with children 3 years of age and older.

SPEECH PATTERNS CONTRAST TEST

The Speech Patterns Contrast ([SPAC] Boothroyd, 1984, 1987) is a 4-alternative, forced-choice test of speech perception originally designed as a research tool to measure the perception of speech contrasts by hearing-impaired children with different degrees of hearing loss. The test measures 4 suprasegmental and 8 segmental contrasts, including location of stress, sex of speaker, presence or absence of pitch variation, direction of pitch change, vowel height and vowel place, presence or absence of voicing of initial and final consonants, continuance versus stop plosion of initial and final consonants, and place of articulation of initial and final consonants. The SPAC requires that the child be able to read the response alternatives, so it is useful only for older children. Boothroyd concluded that although as a group, children with less hearing loss had better speech-perception skills than those with greater hearing loss, it was not possible to predict an individual child's speech perception based on the pure-tone audiogram alone. A number of different factors affect speech perception abilities, and each individual must be evaluated to determine her or his skills. Tests like the SPAC can provide much more specific information than the more global tests that are commonly used. By obtaining the specific information that is available with the SPAC, it is possible to determine the specific auditory skills that an individual possesses and design a therapy program to advance those skills.

Open-Set Word-Recognition Tests

NU-CHIPS OR WIPI WORDS WITHOUT PICTURES

The vocabulary used in the NU-CHIPS is at the three-year-old-level and the vocabulary used in the WIPI is at the three-and-one-half-year-old level. Both of these tests' word lists are excellent for evaluating young children who can perform using an open-set format. The vocabulary level makes them good choices for open-set testing of very young children. Recorded versions of these tests are available.

PHONETICALLY BALANCED KINDERGARTEN LIST

The Phonetically Balanced Kindergarten ([PBK] Haskins, 1949) are 50-item, phonemically balanced monosyllabic word lists selected from the spoken vocabulary of normally hearing kindergarten children. Research by Sanderson-Leepa and Rintelman (1976) has demonstrated that the test should not be used for children younger than kindergarten age because the vocabulary will be too difficult, resulting in depressed scores. There is a recorded version of this test.

ISOPHONEMIC WORD LISTS

The Isophonemic Word, or AB, (Boothroyd, 1968, 1984), consists of 15 word lists, each containing 10 consonant-vowel-consonant (CVC) words. Each of the lists uses the same 30 phonemes, of which 10 are vowels and 20 are consonants. The test may be presented in a recorded or a monitored, live-voice format, and is presented without a carrier phrase. Subjects are asked to repeat what they hear and are scored on the number of phonemes repeated correctly. As previously discussed, phoneme scoring is an excellent way to determine exactly what perception errors the child is making. Because only 10 words are used, the test is quick to administer and the 30 items scored for each test provide sufficient information to make comparisons between different amplification or competing message conditions.

CONNECTED DISCOURSE OR SENTENCE TESTING

Using a nonstandardized procedure, it is possible to get some impression about a child's ability to understand conversational speech using connected discourse. It is important to interpret these results with caution because context will provide a great deal of information to the child. Connected discourse tracking, developed by De Filippo and Scott (1978), scores the child's ability to repeat back correctly phrases and sentences read by the examiner during a 5-minute period. A standardized, open-set sentence test is included as part of the Minimal Auditory Capabilities Battery ([MAC] Owens, Kessler, Raggio, & Schubert, 1985).

Word-Recognition Tests for Severe and Profound Hearing Loss

AUDITORY NUMBERS TEST

This test (Erber, 1980) was previously discussed as both a speech-reception test and a word-recognition test. It is a closed-set test that assesses vowel perception. (See Closed-Set Word-Recognition Tests: Numbers, earlier in this chapter.)

MONOSYLLABIC, TROCHEE, SPONDEE TEST

The Monosyllabic, Trochee, Spondee Test ([MTS] Erber and Alencewicz, 1976) is a test consisting of 12 words: 4 monosyllables, 4 trochees (2-syllable words with stress on the first syllable), and 4 spondees. All 12 pictures are placed in front of the child, who is asked to point to the picture requested by the examiner. The test is scored in two ways: the percentage of words answered correctly and the percentage of words categorized correctly by stress pattern. For example, if the word presented is a trochee, and the child chooses the wrong trochee, the response will be scored as wrong for the word but as correct for the stress pattern. The test was designed for children over the age of 5 years but can be used for younger children who have a sufficient vocabulary.

GLENDONALD AUDITORY SCREENING PROCEDURE

The Glendonald Auditory Screening Procedure, or GASP, (Erber, 1982) was designed as a closed-set test, one portion of which uses the concept of the MTS. It contains 12 words: 3 monosyllables, 3 trochees, 3 spondees, and 3

Table 9–4. Speech-Perception Tests for Severe and Profound Hearing Loss

Auditory Numbers Test (ANT); Erber, 1980
Monosyllabic Trochee, Spondee Test (MTS); Erber & Alencewicz, 1976
Glendonald Auditory Screening Procedure (GASP); Erber, 1982
Discrimination After Training (DAT); Thelemeir, 1982
Early Speech Perception (ESP); Geers & Moog, 1989
Minimal Auditory Capabilities Battery (MAC); Owens et al, 1985
Test of Auditory Comprehension (TAC); Los Angeles County, 1980
Speech Patterns Contrast Test (SPAC); Boothroyd, 1984; 1987

polysyllables. In addition, it has 10 common, everyday sentences, and a phoneme-detection task. Berliner and Eisenberg (1987) report using it in an open-set format for evaluating children with cochlear implants.

DISCRIMINATION AFTER TRAINING TEST

This test (Thielemeir, 1982) is intended for use with children and adults who are prelingually deaf. The stimulus items are taken from the MTS and proceed through 12 levels of difficulty. The first level requires the use of speechreading and audition to determine whether the child understands the stimulus. Testing evaluates speech detection, gross duration and timing cues, and discrimination of speech-pattern perception. The test is administered with a live voice.

EARLY SPEECH PERCEPTION TEST

The Early Speech Perception (ESP) test (Geers & Moog, 1989; Moog & Geers, 1990) was designed to meet the needs of very young, profoundly hearing-impaired children with limited vocabulary and language skills. The vocabulary is familiar to hearing-impaired children by the age of 6, the words used are easily depicted with pictures, and the test can be administered in less than 1 hour. The test is administered using monitored live voice, first using a combination of vision and audition to be certain that the child has the necessary vocabulary, and then, using audition alone. Part I of the test contains a pattern perception subtest and 2 word-identification subtests. The pattern-perception subtest is adapted from the GASP and uses the same 12 pictures and 4 stress categories. Part II is a 12-item, spondee-identification test, with each item having a different vowel. Part III is a 12-item, monosyllabic word-identification test containing similar words. All words begin with *b* and most end with a plosive. Children who do very well are then tested with the WIPI or the PBK. There is a "low-verbal" version for children who do not have vocabulary sufficient for the standard version that uses real objects instead of pictures, and small sets consisting of two or three objects.

MINIMAL AUDITORY CAPABILITIES BATTERY

This recorded test battery (Owens et al., 1985) is comprised of 13 auditory tests and 1 speechreading test. The tests examine phonemic discrimination, sentence identification, suprasegmental features, identification of environmental sounds, and visual enhancement with and without amplification. Because of the complexity of the test, it provides a great deal of information. It cannot be used with young children.

TEST OF AUDITORY COMPREHENSION

This test TAC (Los Angeles County, 1980) is a closed-set, recorded test that evaluates perception of both environmental sounds and speech. It has 10 subtests, beginning with the ability to perceive the difference between linguistic and nonlinguistic sounds (speech versus a cough), and proceeds to the comprehension of speech in the presence of competing messages. The child responds by pointing to pictures.

SPEECH PATTERNS CONTRAST

The SPAC, previously discussed, is a good test for assessing a variety of speech contrasts in children. (See Closed-Set Word-Recognition Tests earlier in this chapter.)

Evaluation of Speech Perception in Infants

A number of researchers have demonstrated that infants can discriminate between different sounds very early in life (Eimas, 1974; Kuhl & Miller, 1975; Morse, 1972; Eilers, 1977). Eilers, Wilson, & Moore (1977) developed the Visually Reinforced Infant Speech Discrimination paradigm (VRISD). This recorded test requires presentation of two phonemes during a 4-second interval and the child is reinforced using a 3-dimensional toy for a head turn when the sound is changed. Initially, the second stimulus is presented at a higher intensity than the first stimulus. Once the child has learned the task, the intensities are equated. Although this test has been used primarily as a research tool, the potential for using it clinically is very exciting. The VRISD would be especially useful in assessing amplification benefits for infants who cannot yet perform other speech-perception tasks.

Test Conditions for Assessing Speech Perception

Evaluating Monaural Functioning

To assess fully a child's speech-perception abilities, it is necessary to perform several tests under different test conditions. Earphone testing provides information about the child's speech-perception abilities in each ear separately. Separate ear information is important for two reasons. First, it is important for diagnostic reasons to know if the child has equal speech perception in both ears. For example, if, pure-tone testing showed equal hearing in each ear, and speech-perception testing demonstrated significantly different results, further testing would be considered to rule out retrocochlear pathology. From a rehabilitation view, it is useful to have information about auditory perception in each ear with amplification. Such information may provide facts about distortion in the hearing aid signal that is not obvious in other ways, or may indicate that the child is not using hearing in one ear optimally, and suggest the need for auditory training in the poorer-functioning ear alone. If there is concern about retrocochlear pathology, PB-PI functions (Bess & Humes, 1979) can be obtained with any of the word-recognition tests discussed previously.

Earphone testing is usually performed at 40 dB SL or at MCL. Because most speech-perception testing is conducted at what should be comfortably loud levels, testing may not provide information about everyday functioning for a child with impaired hearing. To obtain this information, the child needs to be tested at normal and at soft conversational levels, preferably in soundfield.

Soundfield Evaluation

Every child should have auditory functioning evaluated in soundfield regardless of the basic reason for the evaluation. Even a child with a mild, conductive hearing loss who performs well using earphones at 40 dB SL may have difficulty with word recognition at soft conversational levels or in the presence of competing noise. Figure 9–3 demonstrates test results for just such a child. The information obtained by testing at soft conversational levels and with competing noise will be valuable in helping physicians, parents, classroom teachers, and the children themselves recognize the effect of a mild hearing loss on classroom functioning and in determining when medical treatment is indicated.

Testing should routinely be conducted at normal (50 dB HL) and soft (35 dB HL) conversational levels (Madell, 1990; 1996). If test results are extremely poor at normal levels, they need not be obtained at soft levels. After testing in quiet conditions, testing should be repeated at normal and soft conversational levels in the presence of competing noise. The most useful competing message is recorded speech babble. Because the stimulus is speech, it will be more distracting than speech noise or white noise, and more like the message competition that the child faces every day. Babble with one or two voices will be the most distracting because it is easy to understand the words spoken by one or two people. Twelve-talker babble will be easier to ignore than 1-, 2- or 4-talker babble because it is harder to recognize any individual voice. Four or twelve-talker babble is most commonly used. The choice of a noise stimulus is particularly important when assessing children with auditory processing concerns. Noise testing is usually conducted at +5 or +6 dB S/N. If good results are obtained at that level, testing can be repeated at 0 S/N. For soundfield testing, the child should be seated facing the loudspeaker at 0 degrees azimuth, with the speech stimulus coming from the front speaker. The competing message can be presented from the same loudspeaker, from 180° (directly behind the child) or from 90° on both sides of the child. Speech and noise can also be presented from both loudspeakers. When a child has a unilateral hearing loss, it is useful to test with the loudspeakers at 45° or 90° on each side of the child,

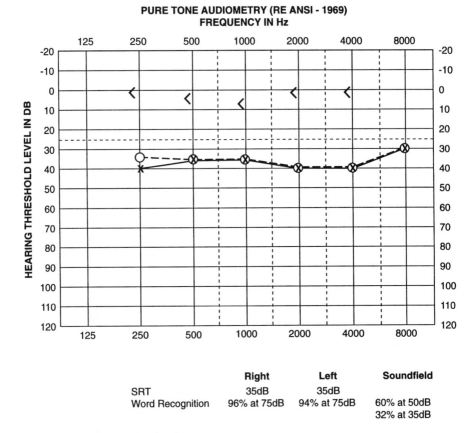

Figure 9–3. Word recognition testing for a child with a mild conductive hearing loss and poor word recognition at normal and soft conversational levels.

with speech directed to the side of the poor ear, and with the competing message directed to the better ear. This will tax the child's auditory capability maximally and make it clear if the child needs assistance, such as a classroom FM system.

A child whose word recognition drops significantly in the presence of competing noise may be demonstrating auditory processing difficulties. Figure 9–4 demonstrates the test results of a child with normal hearing and good word recognition at normal conversational levels, but poor word recognition at soft levels and in the presence of competing noise. Identification of the problem helps the parent, teacher, and child understand that some aberrant academic and behavior patterns do not stem from attention or behavioral problems but rather, from a very real perceptual problem.

Testing with Amplification

The assessment of amplification follows unaided testing, so unaided soundfield test results at normal and soft conversational levels in quiet conditions and in the presence of a competing message will already be available. The same tests should be repeated with amplification. If there is any doubt about the benefit obtained from amplification, this kind of testing should provide the necessary information. If aided test results indicate reduced functioning in quiet conditions or in the presence of a competing message, a good case can be made for the use of FM systems in the classroom and in other situations in which distance from the person talking or competing noise is a factor.

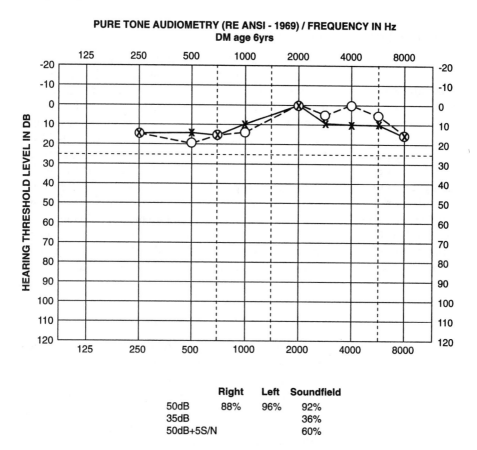

	Right	Left	Soundfield
50dB	88%	96%	92%
35dB			36%
50dB+5S/N			60%

Figure 9–4. Word recognition testing for a child with normal hearing and an auditory processing disorder with good word recognition at a normal conversational level and poor word recognition at a soft conversational level and in competing noise.

Table 9–5. Describing Auditory Function

Unaided vs aided vs FM functioning
Monaural vs binaural functioning
Response to clued vs unclued material
Speech perception at normal conversational levels (50 db HL)
Speech perception at soft conversational levels and at a distance (35 dB)
Speech perception in competing noise
    50 dB HL at +5 S/N
    50 dB HL at 0 S/N
    35 dB HL at 0 S/N
Speech perception with visual cues

Describing Auditory Functioning

A part of each audiological report should include a description of the child's auditory functioning. This report will assist the reader in understanding what to expect from the child in a variety of different situations and will assist the teacher and therapist in planning remediation, if needed. What can you expect from the child when speech is presented at normal and soft conversational levels? What happens in the presence of noise? Can the child perform in an unclued (open-set) situation, or is it necessary for the child to be clued (using a closed set or topic information) to understand? Does the child require paragraph or sentence material to follow conversation or can she or he follow single words? Can the child understand the message on first presentation or does he or she require repetition to understand? If the child wears hearing aids, functioning should be compared when unaided, aided (monaural and binaural), and with an FM system to develop a complete picture of the child's auditory strengths and weaknesses.

Summary

Speech perception testing is an exciting and challenging part of the audiological test battery. By fully assessing speech perception, we are able to obtain valuable information about a child's use of audition that cannot be obtained in any other way. A large variety of speech perception tests are currently available. Combining them appropriately, under a variety of test conditions, allows audiologists to evaluate children of all ages, with all levels of vocabulary, and with all degrees and types and of hearing loss. It provides us with the opportunity to assist in maximizing every child's communication abilities. Speech-perception testing is an essential part of our test battery and in-depth testing should be routinely included in every child's audiological evaluation. By doing so, we fulfill our responsibility to do more than simply identify the presence or absence of hearing loss and do what audiology was intended to do—assess and improve communication function.

References and Readings

American Speech-Language-Hearing Association. (1988). Guidelines for determining threshold level for speech. *ASHA, 3,* 85–89.

Berliner, K.I., & Eisenberg, L.S. (1987). Our experience with cochlear implants: Have we erred in our expectations? *Am J Otol, 8,* 222–229.

Bess, F.B.A., & Humes, L. (1979). Performance intensity functions in cochlear and eighth nerve disorders. *Am J Otolaryngol, 1,* 27–31.

Boothroyd, A. (1968). Developments in speech audiometry. *Sound, 2,* 3–10.

Boothroyd, A. (1984). Auditory perception of speech contrasts by subjects with sensorineural hearing loss. *J Speech Hear Res, 27,* 134–144.

Boothroyd, A. (1987). Perception of speech pattern contrasts via cochlear implants and limited hearing. *Ann Otol Rhinol Laryngol, 96* (Suppl. 128), 58–62.

Boothroyd, A. (1988). Amplitude compression and profound hearing loss. *J Speech Hear Res, 31,* 362–376.

Clopton, B.M., & Silverman, M.S. (1977). Plasticity of binaural interaction: II Critical period and changes in midline response. *J Neurophysiol, 40,* 1275–1280.

Cramer, K.D., & Erber, N.P. (1974). A spondee recognition test for young hearing-impaired children. *J Speech Hear Disord, 39,* 304–311.

De Filippo, C.L., & Scott, B.L. (1978). A method for training and evaluating the reception of ongoing speech. *J Acoust Soc Am, 63,* 1186–1192.

Eilers, R.E. (1977). Context-sensitive perception of naturally produced stop and fricative consonants by infants. *J Acoust Soc Am, 61,* 1321–1336.

Eilers, R.E., Wilson, W.R., & Moore, J.M. (1977). Developmental changes in speech discrimination in infants. *J Speech Hear Res, 70,* 766–780.

Eimas, P.D. (1974). Auditory and linguistic processing of cues for place or articulation by infants. *Percept Psychophys, 16,* 513–521.

Elliot, L., & Katz, D. (1980). *Development of a New Children's Test of Speech Discrimination.* St. Louis: Auditec.

Erber, N.P., & Alencewicz, C.M. (1976). Audiologic evaluation of deaf children. *J Speech Hear Disord, 41,* 256–267.

Erber, N.P. (1979). An approach to evaluating auditory speech perception ability. *Volta Rev, 81,* 16–24.

Erber, N.P. (1980). Use of the Auditory Numbers Test to evaluate speech perception abilities of hearing impaired children. *J Speech Hear Disord, 45,* 527–532.

Erber, N.P. (1982). *Auditory Training.* Washington, DC: A.G. Bell.

Friel-Patti, S., Finitzo-Hieber, T., Conti, G., & Brown, K. (1982). Language delay in infants associated with middle ear disease and mild fluctuating hearing impairment. *Pediatr Infect Dis J, 1,* 104–109.

Geers, A., & Moog, J. (1989). Evaluating speech perception skills: Tools for measuring benefits of cochlear implants, tactile aids, and hearing aids. In Owens, E., & D. Kessler (eds.): *Cochlear Implants in Young Deaf Children.* Boston: College Hill.

Jerger, S., & Jerger, J. (1982). Pediatric speech intelligibility test: Performance-intensity characteristics. *Ear Hear, 3,* 325–333.

Kuhl, P.K., & Miller, J.D. (1975). Speech perception in early infancy: Discrimination of speech-sound changes. *J Acoust Soc Am, 58* (Suppl. 1), 566.

Ling, D. (1978). Auditory coding and recoding: An analysis of auditory training procedures for hearing impaired children. In Ross, M., & T. Giolas (eds.): *Auditory Management of Hearing Impaired Children.* Baltimore: University Park Press.

Los Angeles County, Office of the Los Angeles County Superintendent of Schools, Audiology Services, and Southwest School for the Hearing Impaired (1980). *Test of Auditory Comprehension.* North Hollywood: Forworks.

Madell, J.R. (1990). Audiological evaluation. In Ross, M. (ed.): *Hearing-Impaired Children in the Mainstream*. Parkton, MD: York Press.

Madell, J.R. (1992). FM systems as primary amplification for children with profound hearing loss. *Ear Hear, 13*, 102–107.

Madell, J.R. (1996). Speech audiometry for children. In Gerber, S.E. (ed.): *The Handbook of Pediatric Audiology*. (pp. 84–103). Washington, DC: Gallaudet University Press.

Moog, J., & Geers, A. (1990). *Early Speech Perception Test for Profoundly Hearing-Impaired Children*. St. Louis: Central Institute for the Deaf.

Morse, P.A. (1972). The discrimination of speech and non-speech stimuli in early infancy. *J Exp Child Psychol, 14*, 477–492.

Owens, E., Kessler, D.K., Raggio, M.W., & Schubert, E.D. (1985). Analysis and revision of the Minimal Auditory Capabilities (MAC) Battery. *Ear Hear, 6*, 280–290.

Ross, M., & Giolas, T.G. (1978). *Auditory Management of Hearing-Impaired Children: Principles and Prerequisites for Intervention*. Baltimore: University Park Press.

Ross, M. & Lerman, J. (1970). A picture identification test for hearing impaired children. *J Speech Hear Res, 13*, 44–53.

Ross, M., & Randolph, K. (1990). A test of the auditory perception of alphabet letters for hearing impaired children: The APAL test. *Volta Rev, 92*, 237–244.

Sanderson-Leepa, M.E., & Rintelmann, W.F. (1976). Articulation function and test-retest performance of normal-learning children on three speech discrimination tests: WIPI, PBK 50, and NU auditory test No. 6. *J Speech Hear Disord, 41*, 503–519.

Siegenthaler, B., & Haspiel, G. (1966). Development of two standardized measures of hearing for speech by children (Cooperative Research Program Project #2372). Washington, DC: U.S. Office of Education.

Thielemeir, M.A. (1982). *Discrimination After Training Test*. Los Angeles: House Ear Institute.

Wallace, I.F., Gravel, J.S., McCarton, C.M., & Ruben, R.J. (1988). Otitis media and language development at 1 year of age. *J Speech Hear Disord, 54*, 245–251.

10

The Amplification Evaluation

Selection of amplification is one of the most critical issues affecting the hearing-impaired child. Regardless of the educational system selected by the family, there is agreement that every child should be given the opportunity to make maximum use of residual hearing. This is not a new philosophy. As early as 1884, E. M. Gallaudet and others recognized that hearing-impaired children could benefit from a program that stimulated their residual hearing. Max Goldstein, founder of Central Institute for the Deaf, in 1939 published *The Acoustic Method,* describing a technique for teaching children to use residual hearing based on the training he had received in Vienna in the late 1800s. Ross (1996) reports that in *The Volta Review* alone there were 39 articles published before World War II devoted to stimulating residual hearing with auditory training. By 1936, the majority of schools for the deaf reported using auditory training systems to access residual hearing (Watson & Watson, 1937).

Beginning in the 1920s and 1930s advances in technology made it possible to provide amplification that could be used outside of school so that hearing-impaired children could be amplified during all their waking hours, not just when they were in school. Early amplification was, of course, much more limited than that available today and was more difficult to fit. By today's standards, the hearing aids were large (batteries and amplifiers were in separate packs that had to be strapped to the body), and the quality of the sound was much poorer by comparison. Still, amplification was recognized as extremely valuable in providing hearing-impaired children with access to auditory information unavailable in any other way. The value of audition for language and academic learning and for communication was clearly understood. However, the state of amplification available at that time limited who could use it. Children with severe and profound hearing losses received limited benefit. With the current state of technology, it is now possible to provide adequate amplification to almost every hearing-impaired child, and it is our responsibility as audiologists to be vigilant and aggressive in selecting amplification that truly maximizes auditory access for every hearing-impaired child we see.

Amplification Goals

Obviously, we want to provide the best amplification to every child. But what is the best amplification? How do we decide who needs amplification? How good is good enough? What are our amplification goals?

Who Needs Amplification?

No one would question fitting amplification on a child with a 50- or 60-dB sensorineural hearing loss. That one is simple. However, there are other situations, that are a little less clear. Is amplification necessary for a child (a) with borderline normal hearing (thresholds at 25 dB), (b) with fluctuating hearing loss (fluctuating between normal hearing and 40 dB) secondary to middle ear disease, (c) who does not alert to sound or understand even the most simple speech perception tasks (e.g., vowel discrimination) and who has been wearing amplification, (d) with an auditory processing disorder, (e) with auditory learning disabilities, or (f) with severe developmental disabilities?

Borderline-Normal Hearing

If children with borderline-normal hearing are having difficulty hearing speakers at a distance or in the presence of competing noise, amplification should be considered. To determine if the child is hearing soft speech and needs amplification, it is necessary to evaluate the child's auditory perception at normal and soft conversational levels in quiet and in the presence of competing noise. If the child has difficulty in these situations, amplification should be considered. If the child has any additional learning problems, such as a language disorder or developmental delay, we should expect that even borderline-normal hearing or a minimal hearing loss will have a more significant impact on learning, perhaps indicating that we should be more aggressive in recommending amplification than we would for a normally developing child.

Fluctuating Hearing Loss

What about children with fluctuating hearing loss? Any child (or adult, for that matter) who has a 40 dB hearing loss will have difficulty hearing. If the situation is temporary (lasting 1 or 2 weeks) it may not be necessary to do anything about it. However, if the situation is frequent (ear infections 4 to 6 times per year in which hearing is compromised for several weeks during each episode), amplification should be considered because the hearing loss will be educationally compromising.

Profound Hearing Loss with No Response to Sound

The question of amplification fitting for the child with a profound hearing loss who does not use audition to communicate is more difficult. The first question is, how does the child hear with amplification? Does the child have useful aided hearing? Is the child hearing conversational speech? If not, we cannot expect the child to be able to use audition. The first step is to try to provide more amplification so that the child's hearing can be moved into the conversational speech range. If it is not possible to do this with standard amplification, other options include frequency modulation (FM) systems, tactile aids, or cochlear implants. Once the child is receiving sufficient amplification, the question is, does the child have the opportunity to learn to use hearing? A child with a mild, and possibly even a moderate hearing loss, can learn to listen simply by using amplification and being exposed to speech and sound. A child with a severe or a profound hearing loss will not be able to learn to use hearing without training. For a child with a significant hearing loss, amplification is necessary, but not sufficient, for learning to listen. Before discontinuing the use of amplification, attempt to teach the child to use residual hearing. Almost all very young children should be able to learn to use hearing if amplification provides them with sufficient auditory access to speech stimuli. The older a child becomes, the more difficult it will be to learn to listen. If a child cannot use hearing to understand speech, does that mean that she or he should not use amplification? Not necessarily. Amplification may permit the child to alert to sound so he or she can turn and look at the person who is speaking and then receive the message through speechreading, cued speech, or sign; or to receive warnings (such as of an oncoming car). These may be sufficient reasons to use amplification. However, if a child cannot use audition even for alerting, should the child continue to use amplification?

Auditory Learning Problems

Children with auditory processing problems, auditory attention problems, auditory learning disabilities, and other developmental problems may have normal-hearing thresholds, but results of auditory perception testing that indicate significant problems functioning in competing noise or with other degraded auditory signals. Although their thresholds do not indicate hearing problems, we can expect that they will have difficulties hearing and learning in a classroom setting or with noise at home. The use of an FM listening system with no, or very limited, amplification will be of benefit. The transmitter worn by a teacher, parent, or other students will overcome the negative effects of distance and competing noise, and will allow the child to hear as if the speaker were at his or her ear, significantly improving auditory attention and auditory learning. If the child's auditory perception is causing distortion, as in cases of auditory neuropathy (Sininger, Hood, Starr, Berlin, & Picton, 1995; Starr, Picton, Sininger, Hood, & Berlin, 1996) speech may still not be completely clear, but the elements negatively affecting the auditory environment that make perception even more difficult will be better controlled.

How Good Is Good Enough?

Amplification goals vary from child to child and between educational settings. Audiologists should have high expectations for hearing-impaired children that are not limited by the child's degree of hearing loss or educational placement. As we know from publications in the auditory–verbal and cochlear implant literature, children with severe and profound hearing losses are capable of learning to use even small amounts of residual hearing to access speech. Our responsibility as audiologists is to provide the best possible amplification, amplification that is capable of providing the child with access to conversational speech. If the amplification we offer does not provide speech within the range of conversational speech, we cannot expect that the child will be able to use hearing to receive auditory information and language. Ling (1967), Pasco (1978), and others have demonstrated that conversational speech needs to be within the so-called speech banana to be heard. Pasco has shown that a person who hears at the bottom of the speech banana will hear only 10% of conversational speech, whereas the person who hears at the top of the speech banana will hear 90% of conversational speech.

Speech Acoustics

Speech energy covers a broad frequency range. Most of vowel energy is in the low frequencies (60–500 Hz). This accounts for about 60% of the power of speech information, but only 5% of the intelligibility. Consonants have the majority of their energy in the middle and high frequencies (1000–8000 Hz). They carry only 5% of the energy of speech and 60% of the information needed for intelligibility. (Levitt, 1978; Gerber, 1974). There is a 30-dB range from the softest to the loudest speech sounds (for a given talker). Low-frequency information provides information about rhythm and inflection, as well as about perception of vowels and low-frequency consonants. High frequencies provide information for perception of most consonants and are critical for verb tense (talks versus talked) possession (yours, John's), pluralization (book versus books), and contractions (he's, what's, it's). Unfortunately, most hearing-impaired people have poorer high-frequency hearing than low-frequency hearing, so for them to hear high-frequency sounds, hearing aids must provide more high- than low-frequency energy.

A Review of Cases

When evaluating whether a child is receiving sufficient amplification, it is helpful to look at the aided test results plotted on the speech banana to be certain that they are receiving all the information they need (Figure 10–1). If a child's aided audiogram is at 40 dB in the low and middle frequencies and 45 to 50 dB in the mid-high and high frequencies (Figure 10–2), what can we expect this child to hear? The child will probably be able to alert to sound, will have vowel recognition and low-frequency consonant recognition, and will perceive rhythm and inflection when there is no competing noise, but in competing noise he or she may have little or no speech perception. This child cannot be expected to hear mid-high and high-frequency sounds, including high-frequency vowels (such as *i*, as in *ea*ch), will probably have very limited open-set word recognition and will not be able to

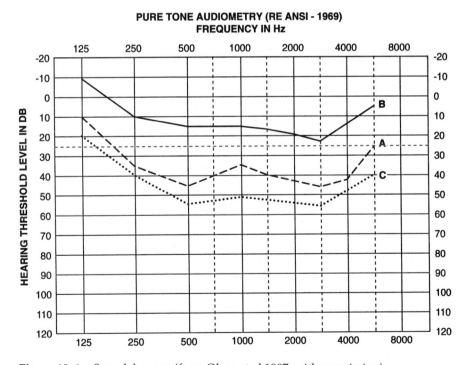

Figure 10–1. Speech banana (from Olsen et al 1987, with permission).

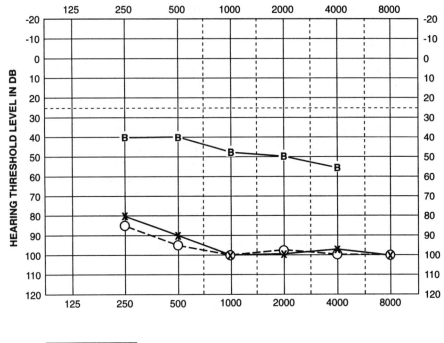

Figure 10–2. Aided audiogram at limits of speech banana in mid-high and high frequencies.

monitor his or her own speech. On the other hand, the child whose aided audiogram is shown in Figure 10–3 can be expected to hear much more. This child hears speech within normal conversational levels for much of the speech range and can be expected to hear most speech sounds. This child will hear best in quiet settings and can be expected to have increased difficulty hearing in competing noise. If this child has been trained to use audition, we would expect her or him to have open-set word recognition in quiet settings and in competing noise, although scores will obviously be

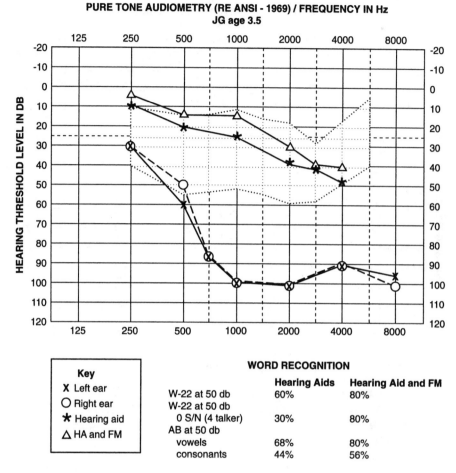

Figure 10–3.   Aided audiogram with aided thresholds within the speech banana throughout the frequency range.

poorer in noise. Figures 10–3, 10–4 and 10–5 demonstrate the advantage provided by a close microphone in an FM system.

Where Does the Child Need to Hear?

One question we need to ask before selecting amplification is, in what situations does the child need to hear? We know that the child needs to hear in school. She or he needs to hear at home, but does the child need to hear as well at home as in school? What about outside on the playground? In the

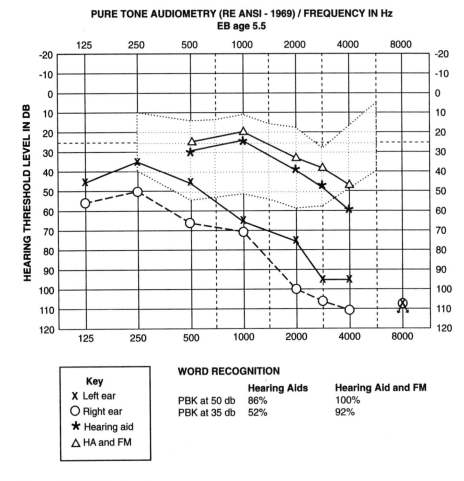

Figure 10–4. FM advantage.

lunchroom? Most audiologists would not recommend fitting a child with a significant hearing loss with amplification only for school. We all recognize the importance of hearing at home. For a preschool child, home is obviously the most critical listening situation because that is where almost all language learning will be done.

Different Amplification Systems for Different Listening Situations?

Should children have different amplification systems for different listening situations? If a child's hearing loss requires an FM system for school use, shouldn't he or she have one for home use? If we think that little learning

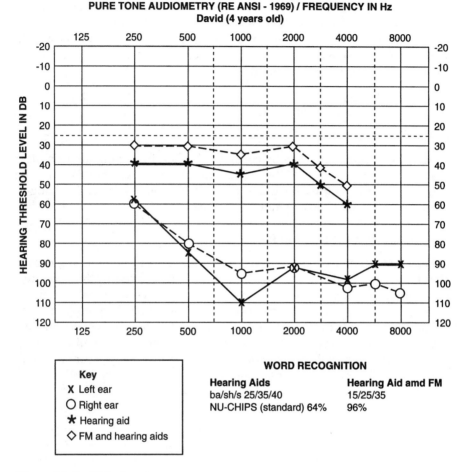

Figure 10–5. FM advantage.

goes on at home, we may not think that an FM system is needed at home. What about the language learning that takes place around the dinner table or while going for a walk or riding in the car? Would an FM system be helpful in those situations? What about the effects of changing amplification during the day? Does changing amplification systems and thus providing different frequency responses or sound quality for different listening situations, cause difficulties in learning for a child who has a hearing loss and for whom auditory perception is, at best, a difficult task?

A good case can be made that children need to be able to hear optimally in all listening situations if they are to learn maximally. Hearing children learn at home, at school, on the playground and so forth; hearing-impaired children need to be able to do the same. There is no reason to believe that a child's home is less noisy then the classroom. Shouldn't the child be able to hear during dinner, while in a car, when watching television? If so, shouldn't an FM system be recommended for home use, too?

Pre-selection Considerations

Initial Considerations

A number of points need to be considered when beginning an amplification evaluation (see Table 10–1). They are all important but may not be equally important for each child at each evaluation. As the child changes, different points will become more or less important.

Degree and Type of Hearing Loss

Every child needs to learn and, therefore, we need to be more aggressive about fitting amplification on children than we would be on adults. Borderline-normal hearing or a mild hearing loss will be educationally compromising, so we know that the child needs amplification for school. The home environment needs to be analyzed. If it is noisy, if there are other children, if the television or radio is frequently on, if the space is small and busy, then amplification will probably be needed for home use, too. Anyone with a moderate or worse hearing loss needs amplification on a full-time basis

Table 10–1. Preselection Considerations
for Selecting Amplification

Primary Considerations
    Degree and type of hearing loss
    Age
    Auditory needs
    Acoustic environment
    Type (style) of amplification
    Monaural vs binaural fitting
    Earmold type
    Child's physical activity level
    Durability of the amplification system
    Repair history of the model being considered
    Ease of manipulation of controls
    FM compatibility
    Safety (locked battery door)
Secondary Considerations
    Cosmetics (size, color)
    Cost

because even a moderate hearing loss causes difficulties hearing in all situations.

The type of hearing loss is not usually a consideration except in rare circumstances, such as atresia. If the hearing loss is permanent, whether it is conductive or sensorineural, it needs to be amplified. A question only arises in the case of fluctuating hearing losses, which are frequently, although not exclusively, conductive. If a hearing loss is present only occasionally, it may not be necessary to provide any assistance. Most people can manage for a week or two. If even short-term hearing loss is a problem, (e.g., if it is very upsetting to the child, or comes at a critical academic time, such as during exam week) some sort of amplification needs to be provided. An FM system with earphones may be sufficient if the loss is mild. If it is more severe, a hearing aid with fitted earmolds may be required.

Age

NEONATES

No infant is ever too young for amplification; in fact, the younger, the better. If we fit amplification early we can significantly reduce the effects of auditory deprivation and bring the child's listening age closer to chronological age. The type of amplification will vary depending on the age of fitting. An infant who is not yet sitting will have problems with a behind-the-ear hearing aid, resulting in feedback when she or he leans back. If the child has a severe or profound hearing loss, a body-worn hearing aid or FM system is appropriate, and will provide sufficient gain and eliminate feedback problems. If the loss is mild, it may still be possible to use a mild-gain, body-worn system until the infant is sitting. If not, special adaptations will need to be made to enable the child to wear hearing aids. If the acoustics can be worked out, a piece of long tubing can be used to attach the hearing aids to a headband or to the child's shirt so the sound does not feed back. If this kind of adaptive system is used, it is critical that it be evaluated electroacoustically because the long tubing will change the frequency response and gain.

INFANTS AND CHILDREN

Once a child is sitting, the choice of amplification style is specifically determined by the child's hearing loss and educational needs, and the auditory environment in which he or she lives. If the child is in an educational environment that emphasizes auditory skills, amplification that provides the most auditory access is critical. For many children, that means full-time use of FM systems.

ADOLESCENTS

Adolescents present their own set of problems, and amplification is the least of them. By the time children reach 12 or 13 years of age, they have very strong opinions about everything and are less easily influenced by adults. At this point, their ears have stopped growing at such a rapid rate. They no longer need earmolds every few months, and there are more amplification options to consider. Self-image is very critical at this time, as is their need to be involved in the selection process of their amplification. This is the age at which children start rejecting FM systems. They do not want to be singled out if they are in a mainstreamed classroom. Children who rely on audition for learning will not give up their hearing aids because they know that they need them to communicate, but they don't want to have to hand a teacher the microphone, pick it up after class, and take it to the next teacher. However, as academic material becomes more difficult, the use of an FM system becomes even more necessary, and ways need to be devised to help the child understand this. It is sometimes necessary to negotiate the use of hearing aids or an FM system, depending on the child's grades. I have negotiated the reinstituting of the FM system previously rejected by an adolescent after her grades started dropping. This is when adolescents begin to consider in-the-ear (ITE) hearing aids. If they can provide sufficient auditory access, they are fine. However, the use of an FM system for school needs to be considered, and most ITEs are not FM compatible. (See discussion under Type of Amplification later in the chapter.) In some European countries, all hearing aids must have a telephone switch, so all are FM compatible.

Acoustic Environment

The need to evaluate the child's acoustic environment cannot be overstated. Ideally, every hearing-impaired child should be within 3 feet of the person who is speaking, and there should be no competing noise. The most appropriately fit amplification system and the best educational program will provide very little benefit if the speech signal is not accessible because it is embedded in background noise. Even minimal noise in the environment interferes with the signal that the child receives, and the acoustic environment in which a child listens has a significant effect on auditory functioning. Finitzo-Hieber and Tillman (1978), Tillman, Carhart, and Olsen (1970), Bess and McConnell (1981), and others have demonstrated that noise has a significant negative impact on hearing-impaired children, more so than on normally hearing children. Hearing-impaired people may require speech levels to be as much as 20 dB greater than the competing noise signal to optimize speech perception.

The distance between the listener and the speaker also has a significant impact on speech perception, especially when combined with noise. In an average ambient-noise environment of 60 dBSPL, average speech at 3 feet will be about 66 dBSPL and the signal-to-noise (S/N) ratio will be +6 dB. If the speaker is 6 feet away, speech will be heard at 60 dBSPL and the S/N ratio will be 0 dB. If the speaker is 12 feet away, speech will be 54 dB SPL and the S/N ratio will be −6 dB. (This is a difficult listening situation for a normally hearing person, but not an unusual one for a classroom.) However, if the speaker were 4½ inches from the listener (accomplished by having the speaker sitting next to the listener or using a close microphone) the speech signal would be 84 dBSPL and the S/N ratio +24 dB. (Ross, Brackett, & Maxon, 1982).

In an ideal listening environment, only one person should be speaking at a time. Windows should be closed if they face street traffic. Noise sources, which include air conditioners, humming refrigerators, dishwashers, TV, and running water, should be eliminated. Human-produced sounds such as walking feet, side conversations, and the moving of chairs should also be eliminated. The chances of ridding the environment of all of these is obviously very close to zero and, in fact, we would not really want to eliminate all sound from the world, but we do want to try to control what we can so that we can make listening and communication as easy as possible for hearing-impaired children and for normally hearing children in a classroom. Carpeting, acoustic tile, and drapes should be used whenever possible. Even a small area rug bought at a remnant sale can do wonders at controlling noise if placed in the block corner. Chairs and tables should have rubber feet so that when they do move, they make only minimal sounds. Noise does not really help anyone hear and normally hearing children in the classroom will also benefit from efforts made to control the auditory environment.

Virtually every hearing-impaired child needs an FM system for school use. No matter how well designed a classroom is, it has a lot of people in it. Children can be noisy, paper and feet make noise. No matter where you are sitting, you are probably at more than the optimal listening distance of 3 feet from the speaker, and the speaker is frequently not facing you. Homes are also noisy. There are frequently other children in them who make noise, toys make noise, appliances and television make noise, and, after infancy when children may be held in someone's arms for a significant part of the day, most children will be at more than the ideal listening distance from the person who is speaking. If we believe that learning takes place at home, we need to make every attempt to control the listening environment at home, too. This frequently means that an FM system should be used at home for at least part of each day. Many parents who use an FM system at home report that they find that having the microphone around their neck encourages them to talk more, which provides more language stimulation to the child.

Educational Environment

Different educational environments have different auditory needs. Mainstreamed children who go to school without interpreters (oral, cued speech, or sign) have the most critical need for optimal auditory skills. In addition to standard amplification, they will need an FM system with a transmitter that is used by every teacher and, hopefully, will also be used by the other children during classroom discussion.

At the other end of the spectrum, children in a self-contained classroom will easily accept amplification because everyone else in the room does. Still, each child hears differently and has different auditory skills. The same hearing aid or FM system is not best for every child, and each system must be evaluated on the child before it is used to be certain it is providing the expected benefit.

Children who use interpreters in class have a more complicated auditory situation. Someone is speaking and the interpreter is interpreting what was said, usually with a time lag. Who should be using the transmitter? If the teacher wears it, the auditory message will be not be timed with the interpreted message. Ideally, the interpreter should be using the transmitter and presenting both the auditory and interpreted message (cued speech, oral, or sign) at the same time. The problem with this method is that the interpreter then must use his or her voice, which may interfere with classroom activities. An additional problem will be encountered with a sign-language interpreter using American Sign Language. Because the sentence structure is different between the two messages, the interpreter may have a hard time speaking standard English and signing American Sign Language. This problem will obviously not exist if the sign language system is Signed Exact English.

Type of Amplification

Almost without exception, people prefer to have the smallest possible hearing aid, as attested to by the demand for in-the-canal (ITC) and ITE aids. All things being equal, children should be fitted with small aids if possible, but only if we can be certain that they are receiving sufficient acoustical information. Size should not be the first consideration.

BEHIND-THE-EAR (BTE) HEARING AIDS

A behind-the-ear (BTE) hearing aid is considered the system of choice for most children, but we should not assume in advance that a BTE will always be so. For the most part, BTE aids are fairly durable and easy to manipulate. Even young children can learn to insert them with ease. Ear-level microphones provide increased ability to localize. There are some very small models that fit well behind tiny ears. A frequent and serious problem with BTE hearing aids for young children is acoustic feedback. The problem is caused by the very small distance between the ear canal and the hearing aid microphone and because the cartilege in the pinna is still so soft that sound radiates through it. The problem becomes worse when we try some of the earmold adaptions, such as horned earmolds. The additional high-frequency information makes feedback even more difficult to control. A very tight-fitting earmold with thick-walled tubing will solve the problem for some children, but not for all. Because most people cannot stand the sound of feedback, especially when it is present almost all the time, the volume control on hearing aid is frequently turned down. Although this reduces the feedback, it also reduces the auditory information received. The audiologist has selected a particular hearing aid and hearing aid setting to provide a certain acoustic signal. If feedback causes the hearing aid to be turned down, the child will not get the same signal. This is a problem for every child (and every person), but especially for children using audition for learning.

BODY-WORN AMPLIFICATION

Infants and young children with profound hearing loss, and many with severe hearing loss, will not receive sufficient auditory information for speech perception with BTE hearing aids. A BTE may not provide sufficient gain and, if it does, the feedback problems will be ongoing. Body-worn systems frequently provide more gain and power. First of all, they are designed to provide greater gain. In addition, because the hearing aid microphone is worn on the chest and not at the ear, the distance from the hearing aid microphone to the earmold will decrease the feedback problem, thereby permitting the child to wear the amplification at the recommended use setting (Ross & Madell, 1988).

Body-worn systems are also very useful for children with physical disabilities who cannot manipulate a BTE hearing aid. The ability to manipulate the hearing aid gives the child control of the amplification, which is important. Giving the child responsibility for managing the amplification will help the child learn to use audition better.

IN-THE-EAR (ITE) AND IN-THE-CANAL (ITC) HEARING AIDS

ITE and ITC hearing aids are very popular with adults and have many advantages. They are small and less visible, and the location in the ear canal takes advantage of pinna effects. However, they also have disadvantages. The fact that they are small makes them easy to lose, and this is a particular problem for children. These hearing aids cannot always provide optimal frequency response, gain, and output, especially for children with very significant hearing losses. Feedback is a particular problem with children who wear ITEs. Another problem is the inability to provide loaner aids. When the hearing aid needs repair or the case needs to be remade because the ear has grown, the child will be without amplification because ITE loaners are not available. But most important, these aids are usually not FM compatible. Some have a telephone coil but this significantly changes the frequency response. Especially in the child's early years, this may be a problem. Once children reach adolescence, when appearance becomes more of a concern, and they have a solid language base, an ITE or ITC hearing aid may be a good choice for use outside of school when an FM system is less critical.

FM SYSTEMS

Virtually every child needs an FM system sometimes; many need one full time. A number of authors have recommended FM systems as primary amplification for children with severe and profound hearing loss (Benoit, 1989; Madell, 1992a and b, 1996; Ross, 1992; Vaughn, Lightfoot, & Teter, 1988). FM systems are important, especially for young children who are trying to learn language and for whom auditory access is critical. The difficulties caused by noise, distance, and reverberation are well known. The advantages offered by use of a close microphone in reducing these effects are also well known. Now that FM amplification is available in BTE casings, cosmetic concerns are no longer an issue, so FM systems are being recommended more frequently.

A variety of different FM amplification styles are available (Madell & Sandrock, 1997). They each have advantages and disadvantages. FM systems can be divided into two categories: those with internal hearing aids and FM receivers, and those only with FM receivers.

Systems with hearing aids come in a variety of models. Body-worn systems with button transducers (Figure 10–6) are excellent for infants and small children with severe and profound hearing loss because they permit the most gain and broadest frequency response without feedback. They also

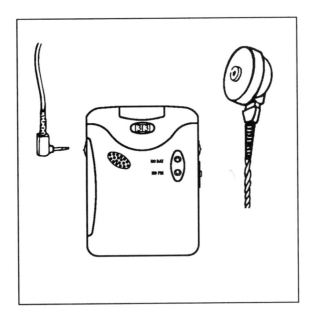

Figure 10–6. Body-worn FM system with button transducers. (Courtesy of Phonic Ear, Inc.)

permit the child to learn to set the controls and to manage amplification independently. These systems also work well for children with physical disabilities who cannot handle smaller systems. The body aid should be worn in a harness or pocket on the child's chest about 4 to 6 inches below the mouth because the child will need to hear his or her own voice through the hearing-aid microphones on the FM system (Figure 10–7). Body-worn systems with BTE ear microphones (Figure 10–8) provide the advantages of hearing at ear level, including localization of sound, but they have the same problems with acoustic feedback that are found with BTE hearing aids. Bone conduction vibrators can be substituted for button transducers for children who cannot wear standard earmolds.

BTE hearing aid/FM systems (Figure 10–9) have become available in the last few years and have made a major change in dispensing practices for children. They offer the cosmetic advantage of a BTE hearing aid and the acoustic advantage of FM systems. The models currently available do not provide the same output and gain as body-worn models, so they may not be the best system for infants and children with severe and profound hearing losses. Two manufacturers have developed FM receivers that are built into an audio-input boot. The advantage of this system is that it permits the transformation of BTE hearing aids into hearing aid/FM systems. When the boot is not needed, it can easily be removed. Because the boot is small

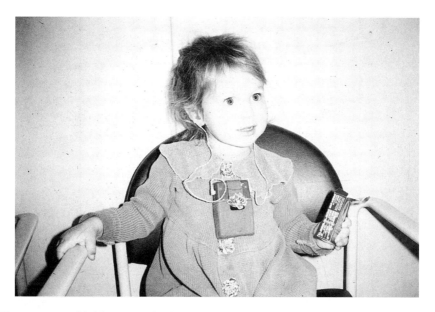

Figure 10–7.   Child wearing body-worn FM system.

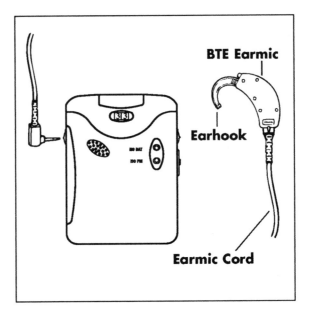

Figure 10–8. Body-worn FM with BTE mic. (Courtesy of Phonic Ear, Inc.)

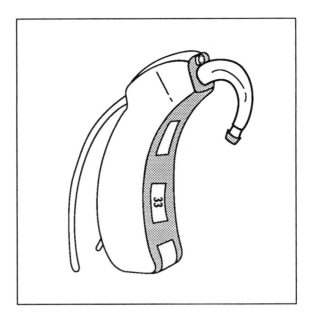

Figure 10–9. Behind-the-ear hearing aid/FM system. (Courtesy of Phonic Ear, Inc.)

and expensive, it should only be recommended to children who are capable of handling it without losing it.

FM receivers without internal hearing aids are for use by children who have personal hearing aids and need FM systems for part-time use. The FM system is in a body-aid case that can be worn in a pocket or on the belt. It can be coupled to the hearing aid either by *direct audio input (DAI)* (Figure 10–10) or with an induction loop (Figure 10–11). DAI coupling uses an audio input boot attached to the hearing aid and a cord connecting the boot with the FM receiver. DAI coupling permits the user to maintain the acoustic signal of his or her own hearing aid. *Induction loop coupling* uses an induction loop worn around the neck attached by a wire to the FM receiver. The frequency response and gain of the induction loop is often significantly altered and the output will vary in response to changes in head and neck loop orientation. It is also be affected by fluorescent lights, computer monitors, and other forms of electrical interference. The hearing aid must be in the telecoil position to receive a signal from the neck loop. If the aid has an Mic–Telephone (M-T) switch the listener will be able to hear her or his own voice as well as the FM signal. However, if the aid only has an M or a T position, the listener will have to select either hearing aid microphone or FM signal. This is not a good choice. Induction loop systems should only be fitted with hearing aids that have M–T switches.

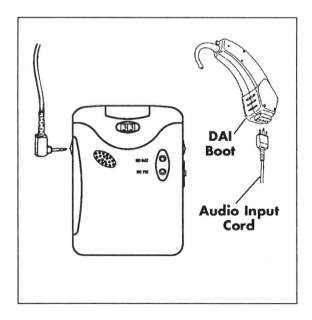

Figure 10–10.   FM with direct audio-input. (Courtesy of Phonic Ear, Inc.)

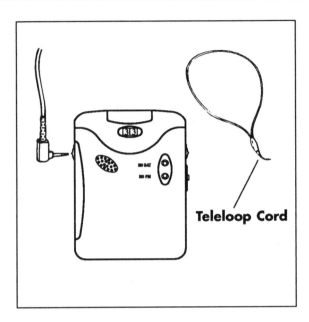

Figure 10–11. FM with (induction) teleloop. (Courtesy of Phonic Ear, Inc.)

Low-gain/low-output FM systems are used for children who would benefit from a close talking microphone but who do not need amplification; this includes children with learning disabilities, auditory processing problems, and difficulties with auditory attention. These systems are available in body-worn, ear-level, and soundfield versions. For the soundfield version, loudspeakers are placed around the room and the signal is available for everyone in the room (Figure 10–12). The body-worn systems are worn with earphones or earbuds. The ear-level versions are in BTE hearing aid cases.

TRANSPOSITION HEARING AIDS

Transposition hearing aids attempt to solve the problems caused by profound hearing loss in selecting amplification. Many children with severe and profound hearing losses do not have sufficient residual hearing for optimal speech intelligibility. One solution is to shift some of the high-frequency energy into lower-frequency regions where hearing-impaired children usually have more hearing. Transposer hearing aids were first developed in Sweden in the early 1960s and were specifically designed to provide high-frequency information in lower-frequency bands. Comparisons between conventional and transposer hearing aids have mixed results.

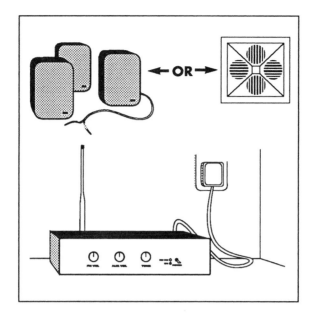

Figure 10–12. Soundfield FM. (Courtesy of Phonic Ear, Inc.)

Two devices are currently available. The Emily and the Transonic are both recommended for people with severe-to-profound hearing losses. The limited information available indicates that children wearing these perform similarly to children with cochlear implants.

COCHLEAR IMPLANTS

A detailed discussion of cochlear implants is beyond the scope of this book. The information needed for the audiologist selecting amplification for children is the knowledge that, should standard amplification not provide sufficient benefit, cochlear implants are available and may be able to provide enough amplification to permit use of audition for language learning. Cochlear implants are recommended only after a trial use of hearing aids. Most of the research indicates that children who are being educated in programs that emphasize use of audition receive the most benefit.

Monaural versus Binaural Fittings

Under most circumstances, binaural amplification is recommended. Two ears permit localization and improve hearing in the presence of competing noise (Hawkins & Yacullo, 1984). There have been several reports suggesting that monaural amplification can have a detrimental effect on speech-perception skills in the unaided ear (Hattori, 1993; Gelfand & Silman, 1993). There are a limited number of listeners for whom binaural listening is not recommended (Madell, 1978a). There are some children (Figure 10–13) for whom binaural word recognition is poorer than word recognition in either ear separately or in the better ear. Before deciding to remove one hearing aid, an effort should be made to train the poorer ear using auditory training tasks with the hearing aid on the poorer ear only. This has been successful in improving auditory skills for some children.

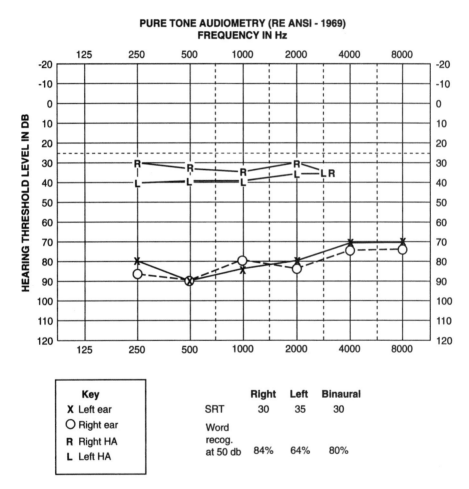

Figure 10–13. Audiogram demonstrating symmetrical aided and unaided hearing with assymmetrical speech-perception abilities.

Earmolds

Selecting an earmold is an important decision. Not only does it need to fit comfortably, it must also be tight enough to eliminate feedback. If the hearing aid cannot provide sufficient gain and output, earmold modification, such as use of horned tubing, can assist in increasing high-frequency gain (Figure 10–14). However, the size of the ear canal will limit the possible acoustic modifications. It does not mean that acoustic modifications should not be tried. If it is not possible for a complete horn to fit in an individual child's ear, it may be possible to fit the child with a modified horn and still receive some increased high-frequency benefit. Unfortunately, using a horn can also can result in increased feedback.

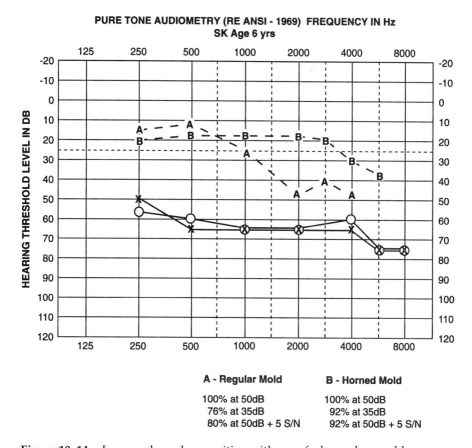

A - Regular Mold	B - Horned Mold
100% at 50dB	100% at 50dB
76% at 35dB	92% at 35dB
80% at 50dB + 5 S/N	92% at 50dB + 5 S/N

Figure 10–14.   Improved word recognition with use of a horned earmold.

If acoustic feedback is a problem, first check that the feedback is not coming from the hearing aid itself, then remake the earmold. If you are certain that the fit is a good one, exchange the earmold tubing for thick-walled tubing. Try use of a distant microphone like a CROS or an FM system, consider a hearing aid with a feedback-suppression circuit or an antifeedback microphone. Every effort needs to be made to find the source of the feedback and reduce it. If we do not reduce the feedback, the volume control of the hearing aid will most likely be turned down, reducing the desired auditory signal.

The color of the earmold and tubing should be considered. If the child is dark-skinned, it might be better to get a brown earmold rather than a pink one. If the child is adventurous, a brightly colored earmold is a good thing to try: They are now available in many colors. By selecting a bright-red, purple, or green earmold a child is saying, "It's okay that I wear hearing aids." This is a very healthy response to a situation the child would like to be able to change.

Physical Activity Concerns

Children should not be limited in physical activity because they have a hearing aid. However, there are some common-sense cautions that need to be observed. If the child is very active and the hearing aid will flop around, the hearing aid may be held in place with tubing or double-faced tape. If the child sweats a lot and the hearing aid cuts off when this happens, it may be worthwhile to try hearing aid "raincoats," which look like small balloons and fit over the hearing aid, or to consider a waterproof or water-resistant hearing aid to be used for sports. Attaching a hearing aid to a sweatband can also occasionally work. Make a hole in the sweatband, and put the body of the hearing aid inside, leaving the tone hook out. This may provide sufficient protection from moisture.

Durability, Repair History, Ease of Manipulation, and Safety

Durability, repair history, and ease of manipulation will eliminate some systems from consideration immediately. Amplification that is recommended for children should be durable: switches should not easily break, the tone hook or FM antenna should be secure, and the battery door should be capable of locking. Controls that we do not want the child to touch should be able to be covered; on the other hand, the controls that need to be accessible should be easy to manipulate. The volume control should not be hidden under something else. The on–off switch should be easily reached. Initially the parents, and then the child, should be able to adjust the controls without much difficulty. For very young children, who might ingest batteries, hearing aids with locked battery doors should be considered.

FM Compatibility

Every hearing-impaired child who is not wearing an FM system as primary amplification needs hearing aids that are FM compatible. At a minimum, the hearing aid recommended for a child should have DAI. Optimally, the aids should have DAI and an M–T switch to permit alternating between different FM options, as needed.

Cosmetic Concerns

If, for a particular family, cosmetic concerns are critical, they will need to be considered, but must always be weighed against auditory factors. For example, if the parents of a 2-year-old child with a profound hearing loss wanted an ITE hearing aid, it would be difficult to justify. It is not likely that we could get sufficient power without feedback to provide access to speech in such a tiny ear. Even if that problem could be solved, as the child grows, the hearing aid will no longer fit and will frequently need to be recased. In young children, this can require recasing as frequently as once every 3 months. During the time the hearing aid is being recased the child will be without amplification since loaners are not available for ITEs.

Cost

It would be nice if cost were not a factor in amplification selection, but unfortunately, it is. Some states, and some counties in some states, provide amplification at no cost to every hearing-impaired child through the Physically Handicapped Children's Program. Many states have financial means tests. Some states will cover hearing aids only, others will provide FM systems. Some states refuse to pay for FM systems, considering them educational devices; others will pay for the receiver but not the transmitter, considering the transmitter educational. Medicaid will purchase hearing aids in most states. Most health insurance companies will not pay for hearing aids unless the hearing loss is the result of an accident or illness. Facilities that treat many hearing-impaired children may receive donated hearing aids or receive funds to purchase hearing aids for children who do not have a source for obtaining them. As health care funding becomes tighter, the cost of hearing aids is clearly a serious problem that will need more attention.

The Amplification Evaluation: The Behavioral Component

After narrowing down the choices, the amplification being considered needs to be tested on the child. Unless it is impossible to do so, the child should have personal earmolds before evaluation. A stock mold or comply mold can do in an emergency, but it will provide a different ear canal resonance and a different acoustic signal than the child's own mold. An amplification evaluation has three parts: electroacoustic analysis of the amplification system, real-ear analysis, and behavioral evaluation. Electroacoustic analysis will provide information about what the output, gain, and distortion of the amplification system is, and real-ear analysis about what signal is reaching the child's eardrum, but neither can tell how the child is using auditory information. Behavioral evaluation is the only way we can obtain this information. Electroacoustic analysis and real-ear analysis are beyond the scope of this book and are well covered in many other books and articles. Some real-ear techniques, such as the Desired Sensation Level (DSL) method was initially designed specifically for the pediatric population and works particularly well (Ross & Seewald, 1988; Seewald, Ross, & Stelmachowicz, 1987). Our emphasis will be on the behavioral component of the amplification evaluation.

The Goal of the Evaluation

There are usually several goals in an evaluation. Obviously, one goal is to determine if the amplification system selected provides sufficient benefit. An equally important goal is to convince the parents, and the child, if she or he is old enough, that the system is providing sufficient benefit. To do this, it is important to compare unaided and aided testing. This is especially important for children with mild or moderate hearing losses. Although you may know that the child is doing much better with amplification, you need to be able to demonstrate it. Begin by obtaining soundfield thresholds in an unaided condition, then proceed to word-recognition testing. The same test stimuli and test conditions will be repeated with amplification. This is frequently a very stressful situation for parents. They do not want to be reminded about how bad their child's hearing loss is but they need to understand the difference between the child's aided and unaided results and what the child can and cannot hear in both situations. The audiological goal of the evaluation is to see that the child is hearing within the speech banana (Figure 10–1), at as high a level as possible, remaining within comfort levels with as wide a dynamic range as possible (not reaching UCLs.) The critical issue is auditory access. Unless the amplification provides enough speech information, the hearing aid will not be useful for speech perception.

Test Room Setup

The test room setup for an amplification evaluation is the same as the one for a hearing evaluation. The child should be positioned as for behavioral testing, preferably seated in a highchair, in the parent's lap, or in an infant seat at the calibrated distance from the speakers. If the child is seated in a highchair or an infant seat, the parent should be off to the side, available to provide comfort, but not too distracting. A test assistant is seated in front of the child and functions in the same way as during a hearing evaluation.

Test Stimuli

FREQUENCY-SPECIFIC STIMULI

Frequency-specific information and speech-perception information need to be obtained. If you have already obtained real-ear testing, you may want to begin with speech-perception testing. If not, begin with warble-tone or noise-band thresholds. This testing will provide information about the contour of the auditory signal the amplification system is presenting although it will only be providing information about soft speech because it is threshold information. If the contour is not what you want, (e.g., insufficient high-frequency information) this is the opportunity to change the settings of the hearing aid or the earmold acoustics. After you have obtained basic frequency-response information, it is necessary to obtain speech-perception information. If the child is not speaking, you may be restricted to speech-awareness thresholds and should get thresholds for low- *(ba* or *bu)*, mid-high- *(sh)* and high- *(s)* frequency stimuli. Many children who are not yet speaking can do picture-pointing tasks.

SPEECH-PERCEPTION TESTING

If the child has speech-perception skills, use whatever test materials are appropriate (see Chapter 9, Speech Audiometry) and obtain speech-perception tests at normal (50 dB HL) and soft (35 dB HL) conversational levels. Regardless of what the child's SRT or pure-tone thresholds are, testing needs to be accomplished at normal conversational levels. The purpose of the evaluation is to see how the child is going to function in the real world, not in a quiet test room with the audiometer set at maximum. If the child cannot hear at a normal conversational level, we may want to try loud speech (65–70 dB HL) to determine if the child has the ability to understand speech using audition but we should not assume that this information will tell us anything about function in the real world. If the child has good or better speech perception for loud levels, it may indicate that the current amplification is not powerful enough. If the child can perform at normal conversational levels, testing should be conducted at soft conversational levels to obtain information about quiet speech or speech at a distance.

Speech perception testing should also be done in the presence of competing noise if the child can perform that task. Four-talker babble is a good stimulus because it is similar to speech in the child's world. Testing should be accomplished at normal and soft conversational levels at +5 S/N. Ideally, this should be set up with the child facing one loudspeaker, with the speech signal and the noise presented from another loudspeaker at 180° behind, or with noise from two loudspeakers at 90°. If only two loudspeakers are available, have the child facing the one from which speech is presented, with noise coming from the other loudspeaker.

If the child uses vision for receipt of information or if auditory skills are very poor, it may be useful to do word-recognition testing with and without visual cues. This type of testing should give you a fairly good impression of how the child will function.

FM Evaluation

Children who use FM systems need to be tested with and without the FM system to determine if the system is providing sufficient benefit. When testing an FM in a soundroom, the child is seated in the calibrated position in the room wearing the FM receiver, and the transmitter is hung 6 inches in front of the loudspeaker, representing the real-use situation when it is 6 inches from the speaker's mouth. When testing speech perception in noise, speech should be presented from the loudspeaker where the transmitter is hung and, noise from the other loudspeaker.

Test Conditions

Although it takes a lot of time, testing should be performed under several test conditions. All testing needs to be done with each hearing aid separately and with both hearing aids together. If the child is using an FM system, testing should be conducted in the hearing aid-only condition (monaurally and binaurally) and with the transmitter. You cannot assume that binaural testing will tell you how a child is hearing in each ear. Only by testing all conditions will it be possible to know how the child is functioning. Figure 10–13 demonstrates test results for a child whose unaided hearing is equal in each ear but whose aided testing showed significantly poorer functioning in one ear. We could not have learned this had we not tested each ear separately. Figure 10–15 demonstrates test results with an FM system in which the transmitter is providing poorer results than the hearing aid condition alone, which should not be the case, and alerts us that something is wrong with the system.

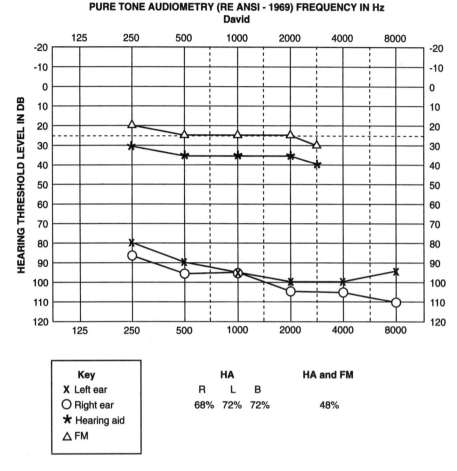

PURE TONE AUDIOMETRY (RE ANSI - 1969) FREQUENCY IN Hz
David

Figure 10–15. Decrease in word recognition with FM system with a broken transmitter.

Fitting Amplification with Minimal Information

Occasionally, audiologists have very little information about a child's functioning. With a very young child, a sick infant, or a developmentally delayed child, it may not be possible to get a complete audiogram in a timely fashion. In some cases, all we have are soundfield thresholds at a few frequencies (500, 2000, and 4000 Hz). Although we certainly need more information, we cannot wait for it before fitting hearing aids. We should obviously begin cautiously, but that does not mean we should not begin. If we cannot obtain separate-ear information because the infant won't accept earphones, or won't respond when wearing earphones, it is possible to obtain separate-ear information with hearing aids by testing each ear separately. If the aided results are the same in each ear, it is probably safe to assume that hearing is similar in both ears. Until you have all the information needed, be conservative in setting gain and output but do not neglect to fit amplification. Every day a child does not hear is a day lost.

How Concerned Should Audiologists Be About Output?

Obviously, we do not want to provide so much output as to cause more hearing loss, but we need to provide sufficient output to provide access to auditory information or there is no point in fitting the child with amplification. The problem of output is usually only a problem for children with severe and profound hearing losses. Children with mild and moderate hearing losses can usually be fitted very well without causing concern about output. There is concern when fitting children with severe and profound losses because output of 132 dB frequently does not bring hearing into the speech range. Although there are reported cases of acoustic trauma in the literature, they are rare. There are also cases of progressive hearing loss with no amplification or with mild amplification. In 30 years of fitting very powerful hearing aids and body-worn FM systems on children with severe and profound hearing loss, I have seen very few cases of drops in hearing, and even fewer that I would attribute to amplification. Let's think about the alternative. We can fit amplification that does not provide the child with access to auditory information but that protects their hearing. How are we benefitting the child if we do this? During critical language-learning years the child will not have access to auditory information. It seems to me that a better choice is to fit as much amplification as is needed and very carefully monitor the child's hearing. Test the child frequently. If the level of hearing appears to be dropping, remove the amplification. If it returns, try again. If it drops again and you believe that the cause is overamplification, then the parents will have to decide how to proceed. The final decision will need to be theirs. The decision is similar to the one faced by parents who are considering cochlear implants. If they have the implant done or fit the child with a very powerful hearing aid that may cause further deterioration in hearing, there may be damage to the hearing of the ear, but by doing so, there will also be in exchange usable auditory function.

Trial Use of Amplification

If at all possible, children should be loaned amplification when the hearing loss is identified and before making a final hearing aid recommendation. This is an expensive recommendation for audiology centers, which will need to have a stock of aids for trial use, but there are several reasons for this suggestion. First, the initial period after identification is a very confusing time for the family. They may be having trouble accepting the diagnosis and need any help we can provide to reduce stress. If we can fit loaner amplification on the child, the immediate pressure of making decisions will be reduced. In addition, as the parents see the child beginning to respond, their stress will be somewhat reduced. Trial amplification is especially useful for children with severe and profound hearing losses. Their access to auditory information has been quite limited, and allowing them to use amplification increases the likelihood of reliable results at the amplification evaluation. As a rule, it is helpful for children to wear amplification for about 3 to 4 weeks before beginning an amplification evaluation.

Helping Families Adjust to Amplification

As difficult as it is to learn that your child has a hearing loss, it is even more difficult to have to face it daily with hearing aids. Until parents recognize the value of hearing aids and see positive responses in their children, they are likely to find them difficult to use. Grandparents will be distressed by it; people on the street look at the child and make sad faces. Before we put hearing aids on, parents may have accepted the fact that their child has a hearing loss, but haven't been confronted by it. They can still be in denial and hope it will go away. A trial with a loaner amplification can help them adjust to their child's hearing loss. Parents don't have to make a decision, and the child can start to be exposed to sound. Parents who are hesitant about having their child wear a body aid or an FM system may be willing to try one on loan because it is not really theirs. Once we can demonstrate to the family that the system works, they are more likely to obtain one. During this period, they can start therapy and meet other families with hearing-impaired children. Parents do not have difficulty accepting body aids or FM systems once they have had the opportunity to see the benefits.

During the initial amplification period, the audiologist needs to be easily available to parents and child. We need to be certain that parents know how to troubleshoot the equipment so that problems are minimal. Because parents will have trouble hearing everything we tell them when we are trying to fit amplfication for the first time, it is helpful to give them printed information to take home (see Appendix 9 for an example of a troubleshooting guide). If the mold is uncomfortable, it may need to be remade several times. If the hearing aid does not fit comfortably on the ear, we need to get a smaller tone hook or a Huggie to keep it in place. If the FM transmitter is causing interference, we should make certain that the parents know how to use it and if that doesn't help, we may need to change the channel to one that has less interference. When I give parents hearing aids, I tell them that they need to be firm about getting their child to accept amplification. They need to remember who is the parent and who is the child. For example, I say, "There are things you do not let your child do. You do not let them run in traffic, you do not let them throw down the lamp in the living room, and you don't let them take off their hearing aids." Parents must realize that they are in control of the situation. At least in the beginning, they need to be the ones to put the hearing aids on and take them off the child. Children learn very quickly that they can get their parents' attention by removing hearing aids. If the child removes the aid, the parent must put it back on. In a short time, the child will understand that the hearing aid is part of his or her body.

Until a child receives a hearing aid, or during a bath or at bedtime when he or she is not wearing hearing aids, parents should be encouraged to speak directly into a child's ear. It is possible to reach 100 dB SPL by speaking with a loud voice, which will provide some auditory stimulation and encourage communication.

Conclusion

Amplification is one of the most critical decisions that will be made for a hearing-impaired child. The audiologist has the opportunity to make a major change in a child's auditory function by carefully selecting and frequently monitoring amplification. Because audiologists see a child only occasionally, they are in a much better position to monitor auditory progress than are the parents, teachers, and therapists who see the child daily or weekly. By providing good access to auditory information and monitoring the child's progress, audiologists can make a significant change in children's lives.

References and Readings

Benoit (1989). House use of FM amplification systems during the early childhood years. *Hear Instrum, 40* 3:8–12.

Bess, F., & McConnell, F., (1981). *Audiology, Education and the Hearing Impaired Child.* St. Louis: Mosby.

Erber, N.P. (1982). Evaluation of special hearing aids for deaf children. *J Speech Hear Disord, 6,* 527–537.

Finitzo-Hieber, T., & Tillman, T. (1978). Room acoustics effects on mono-syllabic word discrimination ability for normal and hearing impaired children. *J Speech Hear Res, 21,* 440–458.

Gelfand, S.A., & Silman, S. (1993). Apparent auditory deprivation in children: Implications of monaural versus binaural amplification. *J Am Acad of Audiol, 4,* 313–318.

Gerber, S. (1974). *Introductory Hearing Science.* Philadelphia: Saunders.

Goldstein, M. (1939). *The Acoustic Method.* St. Louis: Laryngoscope Press.

Hattori, H. (1993). Ear dominance for nonsense-syllable recognition ability in sensorineural hearing-impaired children: Monaural vs binaural amplification. *J Am Acad Audiol, 4,* 319–330.

Hawkins, D.B., & Yacullo, W.S. (1984). Signal-to-noise advantage of binaural hearing aids and directional microphones under different levels of reverberation. *J Speech Hear Disord, 49,* 278–286.

Levitt, H. (1978). The acoustics of speech production. In Ross, M., & Giolas, T.G. (eds.): *Auditory Management of the Hearing Impaired Child.* Baltimore: University Park Press.

Ling, D. (1967). *Speech and the Hearing Impaired Child: Theory and Practice.* Washington, DC: Alexander Graham Bell Association for the Deaf.

Madell, J.R. (1976). Hearing evaluation procedures with children. In Rubin, M. (ed.): *Hearing Aids:Current Developments and Concepts.* Baltimore: University Park Press.

Madell, J.R. (1978a). Amplification for hearing impaired children: basic considerations. *J Commun Disord, 11,* 125–135.

Madell, J.R. (1978b). Hearing aid evaluation procedures for children. *J Acad Rehabil Audiol, 11,* 42–56.

Madell, J.R. (1984). Audiological management of the hearing impaired child in the mainstream setting. *Semin Hear, 5,* 353–365.

Madell, J.R. (1990). Managing classroom amplification. In Ross, M. (ed.): *Mainstreaming Hearing Impaired Children.* Timonium, MD: York Press.

Madell, J.R. (1992a). FM systems for children birth to age five. In Ross, M. (ed.): *FM Auditory Training Systems: Characteristics, Selection, and Use.* Timonium, MD: York Press.

Madell, J.R. (1992b). FM systems as primary amplification for children with profound hearing loss. *Ear Hear, 13,* 102–107.

Madell, J.R. (1996). FM systems: Beyond the classroom. *Hear Instrum, 13,* 30.

Madell, J.R., & Sandrock, C. (1997). Selecting an FM system: When a hearing instrument is not enough. *Hear Rev,* June, 8–16.

Olsen, W.O., Hawkins, D.B., & VanTassel, D.J. (1987). Representation of long-term spectra of speech. *Ear Hear, 8,* suppl, 1005–1085.

Pasco, D.P. (1978). An approach to hearing aid selection. *Hear Instrum, 29,* 12–16.

Ross, M. (1996). Amplification for children: The process begins. In Bess, F.H., Gravel, J.S., & Tharp, A.M. (ed.): *Amplification for Children with Auditory Deficits.* Nashville, TN: Bill Wilkerson Center Press.

Ross, M. (1992). Room acoustics and speech perception. In Ross, M. (ed.): *FM Auditory Training Systems: Characteristics, Selection, and Use.* Timonium, MD: York Press.

Ross, M., Brackett, D., & Maxon, A. (1982). *Hard of Hearing Children in Regular Schools.* Englewood Cliffs, NJ: Prentice-Hall.

Ross, M., & Madell, J.R. (1988). The premature demise of body worn hearing aids. *ASHA, 30,* 29–30.

Ross, M., & Seewald, R.C. (1988). Hearing aid selection and evaluation with young children. In Bess, F.H. (ed.): *Hearing Impairments in Children.* Parkton, MD: York Press.

Seewald, R.C., Ross, M., & Stelmachowicz, P.G. (1987). Selecting and verifying hearing aid performance characteristics for young children. *J Acad Rehabil Audiol, 20,* 25–37.

Sininger, Y.S., Hood, L.J., Starr, A., Berlin, C.I., & Picton, T.W. (1995). Hearing loss due to auditory neuropathy. *Audiol Today, 7,* 10–13.

Starr, A., Picton, T.W., Sininger, Y., Hood, L.J., & Berlin, C.I. (1996). Auditory neuropathy. *Brain, 119,* 741–753.

Tillman, T.W., Carhart, R., & Olsen, W.O. (1970). Hearing aid efficiency in a competing speech situation. *J Speech Hear Res, 13,* 789–811.

Vaughn, G., Lightfoot, R., & Teter, D. (1988). Assistive listening devices and systems (ALDs) enhance the lifestyles of hearing-impaired persons. *Am J Otol,* (Suppl.) *9,* 101–106.

Watson, R.B., & Watson, N.A. (1937). Hearing aids in schools for the deaf. *Volta Rev, 39,* 261–266.

11

Counseling

The Parents' Perspective

Bringing your child for a hearing evaluation is a stressful event: It is stressful the first time the child is evaluated and continues to be stressful for many years to come. A child is brought for evaluation the first time because of concern about the child's auditory status. Parents have probably been worried for a long time by the time they arrive for the child's hearing evaluation, and have probably been testing the child at home to determine how the child hears. From the audiologist's viewpoint the problem may be relatively minor (a temporary conductive hearing loss), or more serious (a permanent sensorineural hearing loss.) The loss may be mild, which from our perspective will cause only minor problems for the child, or it may be severe, having a long-term educational effect. Whatever the diagnosis, it probably could be even worse from the audiologist's viewpoint because, as audiologists, we have seen children who are more severely impaired. From the parents' viewpoint, however, the problem can never be minor and very little could be worse because for them, "Something is wrong with my child!"

Re-evaluations for children already diagnosed with impaired hearing are also very stressful. As many parents have reminded me, every re-evaluation brings up all the parents' old fears and emotions. It is an enforced reminder that their child has a hearing loss, and it causes them to face fears about whether the loss has become worse and to assess their child's functioning: "Is my child doing well enough? Will she or he go to college? Will he or she hold down a job?" These fears and concerns are not different than those experienced by all parents, but they are more intense for parents of a child with a disability. During daily activities parents can usually manage to put them out of their minds, but coming for an evaluation usually brings their fears and concerns all back.

When Counseling Begins

Counseling begins when an audiologist first meets the family in the waiting room. The way we present ourselves tells the family a lot about who we are. Do we introduce ourselves very formally, indicating that we are in charge, or more casually, indicating that we are partners in the evaluation experience? Do we talk to the child and try to make both child and parents comfortable? Are we smiling or stern? Do we conduct all our business standing up, indicating that time is limited and that we can only spend a few minutes with them, or do we sit down next to the parents (not behind a desk) and make the parents feel that we will take the time to understand their concerns and answer their questions? How do we begin talking with the family? It is sometimes helpful to start by asking how they are and, if they seem distressed, acknowledge that we understand that this is a very difficult time. Acknowledging their distress can make them feel more at ease. It does not eliminate the distress, but it gives it value.

Counseling continues as we take the history. During this time we find out why the parents are there, what they are concerned about, and what they may be ready to do. When the evaluation has been completed we need to be certain to address the concern that brought the family to the evaluation. The first thing to find out is who requested the appointment. If the parents were concerned about the child's hearing and requested the appointment themselves, they are more likely to be ready to hear that there is a problem. If parents have come because the pediatrician or the grandparents wanted the appointment but do not have any concerns of their own, they will have a much more difficult time accepting test results that indicate that something is wrong. If this is the child's first evaluation, the parents will not know what to expect. Parents (and the audiologist) may guess what testing may confirm, but there is so far no test information. Sometimes parents have sought out several other opinions before coming for the current evaluation. Sometimes they will share this with you, and other times not. I have had parents say, "I have seen two other audiologists but I don't want to show you the test results before you test her yourself." That is a perfectly reasonable request. I have also had parents volunteer that they have had previous evaluations only after I had discussed my test results.

Sometimes each parent feels different about the evaluation. One parent (frequently the mother, who may spend more time with the child) may be concerned and thus seeking evaluation, while the other parent is present but has no real concerns. It is not unusual to hear one parent say, "I think he hears fine but my wife/husband is the nervous type, so we came for a hearing test." When this happens, counseling is difficult because the parents will want and need different things.

It is important that we remember our role. We are here to educate the parents, to provide information, and to help parents make their own decisions. We need to be certain that we are talking in language they understand, not audiology jargon. We provide guidance. Although we may know much more about hearing loss or developmental disabilities than the parent does, they know more about their child and family. This is most important, and we must always remember it. It is they, not we, who will have to live with the consequences of any decision that is made.

The Parents in the Test Situation

Because parents will, in fact, be making treatment and management decisions, they need to have as much information as we can possibly provide. This means that they need to be involved in all testing and testing decisions. Parents should be in the test room during the evaluation. If grandparents are present, they should be invited in, too, if there is enough room. If not, they may be able to observe testing by sitting with the audiologist and looking through the test-room window. Every effort should be made to find a way to have the parent observe testing, especially if the parent has any question about the presence of hearing loss. If the parents cannot observe, it will be difficult for them to understand test results and make appropriate decisions.

In addition to needing to observe testing, parents can be very helpful in the test room. They may be able to get the child to cooperate when you cannot. They can calm a distressed child and encourage cooperation. Parents will be most helpful in the test room if they understand what is going on. The audiologist should explain the test task—observation, visual reinforcement, or play. Tell the parents what you will be doing, what you expect of the child, and of them. If you have any question about whether the child will be able to perform the task, ask the parent. If the parent volunteers that the child won't be able to perform the task but you believe that the child may be able to do it, suggest that you try but will change the task if the child cannot do it.

Occasionally, a parent is too distracting and interferes with testing, for example, by telling the child to respond when the parent hears a sound even though the child has not demonstrated that she or he has heard it, or by discounting testing by saying, *"He is not interested in this," "The toys are boring,"* or *"He just doesn't want to pay attention."* If that happens, the audiologist needs to help the parent see the difference between not hearing and not responding. Sometimes, it helps to ask the parent just to observe. If you tell the parent to do so, you need to explain why you are doing it so that the parent understands that you are trying to improve the test results, not discounting them or their opinions.

Discussing Test Results

The first step in discussing test results is to explain what happened in the test room. State the facts. Describe what you did and what you observed. Ask the parents what they thought about the testing. Did they think it was a good test? Did they feel the child was cooperative? Let the parents direct the way to proceed. Using an audiogram, show where we expect children with normal hearing to respond and where their child responded. An audiogram that shows familiar sounds and speech sounds (see Appendix 5) can help parents develop a little perspective about what the hearing loss means. Explain what you know and what you do not know. If you did not use earphones, explain that you do not know what hearing is like in each ear. The audiologist needs to determine what the parent can accept. If the parent has normal hearing and heard sounds the child didn't hear, it will be difficult for them to deny the test results. Parents may question whether children hear at the same levels as adults do, whether attention was a factor, or whether the toys were too distracting. We must be prepared to answer these questions. If a child has a sloping audiogram and responds to some sounds and speech but not to other sounds, we need to explain how this will affect speech, language, and academic development.

If the parent is not ready to accept the results, you cannot proceed. You can only proceed as quickly as the parents can go. Suggest a re-evaluation as quickly as the parent is ready to proceed. Ask if the parents would like to seek another opinion, and make it clear that you will not be insulted if they do. Suggest that between this appointment and the re-evaluation, the parents observe and record what sounds the child hears when there are no clues, what words he or she understands, and what directions the child can follow without gesture or situational cues. It is important that the parents feel that you are accepting their opinion and are respectful of their views. In fact, if you do not respect their views, the parents will probably sense your annoyance or disapproval and it is not likely that you will be able to develop a respectful working relationship with them.

Once you have told parents that you believe that their child has a hearing loss, it is likely that they will not hear or retain much else. No matter how prepared they think they are for the information, it is a shock. If they appear confused, ask if they want to stop and discuss it later. Offer paper and a pen to take notes. Although every parent reacts differently, we can assume that all parents are disappointed and distressed by such news. Whatever they imagined for themselves and their child during the pregnancy and until the time of the diagnosis must now change. It doesn't mean that the child will not be loved and wanted, but their dream of a certain kind of child and their expectations for that child's life and for themselves is lost. Audiologists need to recognize this and accept the parents' grief.

Providing Information

Some parents are not capable of taking anything away from the initial evaluation and audiologists need to accept that. Although the value of early identification is apparent, nothing terrible will happen if the child waits an additional 2 weeks to receive services. When the parent is ready for information, we need to be prepared to provide resources. The basic information that needs to be shared is (a) a description of the hearing loss, (b) habilitation/educational options, (c) amplification options, and (d) resources for additional information.

We need to provide this information in as objective a fashion as possible. Parents of a child with a severe or profound hearing loss need to know that there are differences of opinion about educating hearing-impaired children and they need to be encouraged to learn about all of them before making a decision for their child. They need to understand that there are different amplification options and that each has positive and negative features. Regardless of the educational option the parents select, the child will need amplification, so while parents are learning about educational options, they can begin the amplification process. For many parents, the need to do something immediately is critical. Amplification is a good place to begin. Some parents will want to move quickly and will be prepared to let you take earmold impressions the same day the hearing loss is diagnosed. Other parents are stunned by the diagnosis and need a little time to adjust before moving on to the next step. It may be better if you make an appointment to take earmold impressions in a few days or a week to allow the information to sink in. When the parents return for earmold impressions, they may be better able to ask questions and to hear your explanations.

Because it is so difficult for parents to retain information provided at early counseling sessions, it may be helpful to provide written information. It is useful to have a selection of materials that can be provided to parents. These materials might include the following: (a) basic description of hearing loss, (b) a description of educational options, (c) a description of amplification options, (d) resources for additional information, (e) information and resources on different communication modes, (f) financial information for obtaining therapy and amplification, (g) contact list of other parents with hearing impaired children, and (h) information about parent support groups (see Appendices 5–10, 13 and 14).

The audiologist can select any or all of the information pieces to provide to parents. The materials can be taken home to be read over and over until they are understood (see Appendix for examples of handouts). It will be helpful to the parents if we either tape the interview for them to take home or speedily send them a written summary, so they can review what was said. It is very likely that many questions will come to mind after they leave the office, and parents should be encouraged to get a notebook to write down concerns and questions to discuss at the next visit. If the next visit is a long way off and they feel they cannot wait, they should be given permission to call. We need to be clear that we are available to help them. There should be some time each day, or a few days each week, when audiologists are available by phone. Answering questions as they come up will make life easier for the parents and, by extension, for the audiologist. If they abuse this availability and start calling on a daily basis with noncritical issues, they can be asked to write their questions down for discussion at the next visit. Calls to discuss noncritical issues sometimes are really about other concerns; it may be helpful for the audiologist to try to find out what those concerns are.

Providing Emotional Support

Having your child diagnosed with a significant disability is distressing for every parent. All will go through a period of grief or mourning when a disability is diagnosed. Initially, they are in shock. As the shock lessens they begin to feel anger, sadness, and sometimes, denial; they also frequently feel guilt, blame, disappointment, confusion, and helplessness. Eventually, these feelings decrease and parents reach acceptance and recognition, although many say the pain never completely disappears. Different people spend different amounts of time in each stage of grief; many parents move back and forth between stages. They move forward, and then when something changes, (a change in hearing levels, amplification, school setting, a birthday party) earlier feelings resurface. As audiologists, we need to recognize the stages of grief and be aware of how they affect the parents and child. Frequently they are angry and may react angrily to the audiologist or other members of the clinic staff. It is usually not us with whom they are really angry but we are a convenient way to let it out. Audiologists need to acknowledge their anger and frustration but not take it personally. When parents repeatedly come late for appointments, miss appointments, or bring the child without hearing aids or with dead batteries, we know that they are angry and possibly in denial. Getting angry at the parents won't help. It might help to acknowledge the situation by saying something like, "You seem to be having a really hard time. Having a hearing-impaired child is very difficult," thus letting the parents know that we accept the problem without passing judgment. Once we have done this, we increase the possibility that they can accept our assistance.

Some parents need to deal with their grief before being able to attend to their child's needs. Others will refuse to deal with their emotional needs until the child's needs are met. When they are ready, ask if they would like the names of other families to speak with or would like another family to contact them. If there are parent support groups available, invite them to attend. Other parents will be able to provide information and support that audiologists cannot provide. They have been there. We have not.

Coping with a Diagnosis

People cope in different ways. Some people are able to recognize the positive things about their child that are not affected by the diagnosis. Some can count their blessings or seek out support from friends or from other families in the same situation. Some people seek spiritual support through their church or temple, through meditation, or through reading. Some seek out support groups. Others learn as much as they can about the disorder through reading, workshops, and conferences. For others, the diagnosis is overwhelming and there is a need for counseling to get through it.

Initially, many parents express guilt, for example, "Why didn't I recognize this sooner?", "Did I do something while I was pregnant that caused this?", or "Is this because I drank wine on New Year's Eve?" Our role is to provide comfort and information to help parents move forward. Parents want to know what caused the hearing loss. We don't usually know the answer and this fact may be very difficult for them to accept. They need answers and we don't have them. For some parents, this need for information interferes with the ability to move forward. Other parents can provide for their child's needs and work through their grief as they proceed.

Any form of coping is good as long as it does not interfere with providing services for the child. A number of years ago, the mother of a hearing-impaired child with whom I was working told me she had taken her daughter to a faith healer to cure her hearing loss. I was horrified (not the best possible reaction) and expressed my dismay. She, being much wiser than I, said, "Look, as long as I don't take her hearing aids off and continue to take her to therapy and work with her at home, what is wrong with my going to a faith healer?" She was correct. As long as her daughter was getting the help she needed, anything her mother wanted to do to cope was fine. The mother and I still laugh about this 15 years later.

Listening to Parents

A good counselor is genuine in caring about the child and family, honest in providing information and expressing feelings, and a good listener. A good counselor can accept parents' feelings without judgment and recognizes that his or her values and the parents' values may be different. The parents and audiologist may come from different cultures and have different expectations about education, behavior limits, and goals for children.

David Luterman (1979, 1969) says the most important clinical skill we can offer is the ability to listen. We need to be able to listen to parents and to understand what they are saying, acknowledging their feelings whatever they are. Feelings are not good or bad. When a parent expresses concern about something he or she may have done during the pregnancy, we need to recognize the underlying message ("Did I cause the hearing loss?") and respond to it. It is very easy to feel guilty when you have a child with a handicap. We need to listen to parents' concerns. Think about how you would feel if you were very upset and someone just told you not to worry. It would not make you feel better, and it certainly would not make you feel like discussing your problems with that person again. We need to remember this when parents speak to us. Their concerns are not minor, no matter what they are about.

The best help we can offer parents are the skills to solve their problems by themselves and the assurance of our faith in their ability to do so. Empowering parents is the greatest gift we can provide. Listening to parents rather than telling them what to do sends the message that we believe they are capable of making decisions on their own. As Luterman (1995, 1996) reminds us, listening means really listening, not trying to come up with counter-arguments while you are listening. It means putting your views aside and trying to understand without judging. It is one of the most challenging tasks audiologists can try to accomplish.

Who Should Provide Counseling?

The audiologist who is responsible for diagnosis and management of the child's hearing loss has the child as his or her first responsibility. This person provides information to parents and certainly provides support, but other people should be available who have primary responsibility for the supporting parents. This person may be an audiologist, a social worker, a psychologist, or a peer counselor. This person can provide an opportunity for parents to discuss their concerns without judgment and without it interfering with their child's management. If this is not available in the center where the child is receiving services, the child's audiologist should be able to arrange for counseling elsewhere.

Dealing with Angry Parents

It is not unusual for parents to be angry at the audiologist. Audiologists are frequently the bearers of bad news. We tell parents things they did not want to hear and assist them in planning for a life they did not choose. On one level, the parents know that we are not responsible for the fact that their child is hearing impaired but making us angry may be less dangerous than alienating family members. In some cases it is the clerical staff who are recipients of the parents anger. Parents may feel that they don't need something from the clerical staff but will need help from the audiologist, so it is safer to express anger at secretaries. Everyone should realize that this is misplaced anger and try not to take it personally. When a parent yells at us we need to say something like, *"You seem very upset. This must be difficult for you."* This gives the parent the opening to talk about what is troubling them.

On the other hand, sometimes their anger is legitimate and we also need to recognize that. If a child has an appointment at 2 PM and we have not yet seen the child an hour later, the parent may really be distressed. The child may be getting fidgety and the parent may be concerned about another child who will arrive home shortly from school. We might have avoided the anger if someone had informed the parent that the audiologist was late, tied up with another patient, and assured the parent that the audiologist will spend as much time with them as their child needs. Although this won't completely solve the problem for the parent, it assures them that they are not being ignored and that we respect their time commitments, too.

When a parent frequently arrives late for appointments, audiologists can become distressed. We have other patients scheduled and having a family come late can mess up the schedule. It is not productive to become angry at the family. Sometimes parents are late for legitimate reasons: the car broke down, a traffic jam, etc. Sometimes the reasons are not legitimate: there was something else to do which delayed them or they had difficulty getting up in the morning. Sometimes parents are used to clinic appointments where everyone is told to arrive early and are taken in turn. When families are late, we have several options. We can refuse to see the child, we can start the evaluation and complete as much as time allows, or we can turn the family away, which may "teach the parent to come on time," but the person we are really punishing is the child.

Dealing with Other Family Members

In this day and age there are many different versions of family. Some are traditional, nuclear families, but many are not. In some cases there are extended family members who are a part of the child's life and who should be included in our efforts to provide information. If there are siblings who are old enough to understand what is happening, they should be included. The parents must lead the way in determining who should be included and when. We should offer to provide information and counseling to others when needed. If a mother says, "My mother is driving me nuts. She cries every time she sees Lucy with a hearing aid," the audiologist should first acknowledge how difficult this must be for her, then ask why she thinks her mother is reacting this way. Maybe it would be helpful to both of them if grandmother came to the next hearing test or therapy session and learned a little more about hearing loss. It is difficult for parents to accept that the grandparents are going through the same stages of grief that they are. News of the hearing loss often comes at a time in the grandparents' lives when they thought they were done with the difficult aspects of child rearing and expected only the joys of grandparenting. In addition, the grandparents often do not have the advantage of doing something proactive to help the child, as the parents do. If grandparents can provide support, they can be of great assistance, providing respite for parents, assisting with driving to therapy or hearing tests, and, most important, providing emotional support. However, if the grandparents cannot provide support, the parents may need to go it alone for a while.

Siblings need special support. Because the hearing-impaired child requires a lot of attention, the nondisabled sibling sometimes feels left out. Audiologists can be of assistance by reminding parents that siblings need to understand what is happening and need some time alone with the parents. As they get older, they may need to talk about their feelings about having a hearing-impaired sibling. They have to cope with their anger at time taken away from them and guilt at having normal hearing. They need to be monitored so that counseling can be provided, if needed.

Counseling Hearing Impaired Children

When hearing loss is identified, a great deal of time is spent educating the child's family about hearing loss. By the time a child is 7 or 8 years old, the parents know a lot about hearing loss and counseling and hearing testing takes much less time, especially if the hearing loss is stable. By this age, the hearing-impaired child is ready to understand about hearing loss. We need to start to explain the audiogram to the child, to show them what they can and cannot hear with hearing aids, and to give them the opportunity to ask questions. I remember the first time I asked an 8-year-old boy if he had any questions about his hearing loss. He asked when he would be old enough not to need hearing aids anymore. His parents and I were both surprised to realize that he did not understand that his hearing loss was permanent. I recently asked a 12-year-old girl if she had any questions about her hearing loss and she asked why her twin had normal hearing and she did not. It gave her the opportunity to express her anger about the situation and to cry about it. Her parents were very surprised by the strength of her emotions because she had not expressed this to them before.

Hearing-impaired children may need to go through the same grieving process as their parents did when the hearing loss was first identified. It frequently comes as a surprise to the parents because they have usually finished grieving when the child is ready to start. It is also difficult for the child because she or he is grieving alone. Support groups for children are very valuable. It enables them to express feelings and to ask questions of peers, which is something parents and audiologists cannot provide. There are "chat" groups about hearing loss on the Internet for both parents and kids.

The Impact of Diagnosing Hearing Loss on Professional Staff

Each time audiologists diagnosis a child with a hearing loss we, as professionals, may go through a stage of grief that is similar, but less severe, than that experienced by the parents. The first few times are the worst. If we get the opportunity to diagnose hearing loss frequently, it becomes a little less painful but the distress never really disappears. This is good because it permits us to become better counselors and to provide better support for the parents. However, if we, as professionals, see many sad families, and are not feeling hopeful about the future of the children or their parents, our jobs become depressing and eventually we shut ourselves off from the families. We need to pay attention to how we are feeling. If we are shutting ourselves off, we may need a break from working with this population. Many professionals benefit from a support group to assist in dealing with the grief of hearing loss. It may be as simple as eating lunch together once a week to talk about concerns or may require a more structured environment. The more we understand about our feelings, the better we will be at doing our job. Feelings are not good or bad, they just are. We need to remember this as we deal with our feelings and with our patients' feelings.

References and Readings

Atkins, D.V. (1995). Beyond the child: Hearing impairment and the family. *Volta Voices*, September/October, 14–18.

Luterman, D. (1967). A parent-centered program for preschool deaf children. *Volta Rev, 69*, 515–520.

Luterman, D. (1969). Hypothetical Families. *Volta Rev, 71*, 347.

Luterman, D. (1979). *Counseling Parents of Hearing-Impaired Children*. Boston: Little, Brown.

Luterman, D. (1995). Counseling for parents of children with auditory disorders. In *Auditory Disorders in School Children (3rd ed.)*. New York: Thieme.

Mencher, G.T. (1996). Counseling families of hearing-impaired children: Suggestions for the audiologist. In Gerber, S. (ed.): *The Handbook of Pediatric Audiology*. Washington, DC: Gallaudet University Press.

Pieper, E. (1976). Grandparents can help. *Except Parent, 6,* April, 7–11.

Roush, J. & Matkin, N.D. (1994). *Infants and Toddlers with Hearing Loss: Family Centered Assessment and Intervention*. Baltimore: York Press.

12

After the Audiological Evaluation: What Next?

Identification of a hearing loss and the fitting of an amplification system is only the first step in managing a child's hearing loss. Once hearing loss has been identified, the difficult work begins for the child and the family. Professionals from a wide variety of specialties should be available, as needed, to be part of the team for diagnosis and treatment. Individual families and individual children will have different needs and those needs may change over time. Ideally, the team members should work together on a long-term basis. They may be located in the same facility or in independent practices with a loose affiliation. Services may also be located in hospitals, in schools, in community clinics, or in private practices. There are several tracks that the child and family travel along at the same time, moving back and forth between tracks. All evaluations need to be completed to determine if the child has any medical or educational issues that might influence treatment. The family should become informed about educational options and select the one they wish to pursue for their child. The family must select a specific educational program and a management team, and family members must deal with their feelings about hearing loss and about having a hearing-impaired child. Diagnostic services are usually attended to first, but sometimes, during therapy, the need for additional diagnostic services becomes apparent. For example, some children who have middle ear disease, and for whom very little appears to be needed, may require additional diagnostic and treatment services. During therapy it may become apparent that a child with a sensorineural hearing loss has motor problems.

Planning Services

An initial part of the process is to assess a child's communicative competence and the ability of the family to provide assistance to the child in developing communication skills. This is most easily accomplished if the team members and the family have a collaborative attitude. They need to feel that they can work together, share information and opinions with respect, evaluate strengths and weaknesses among the collaborators and the family, share concerns, and acknowledge each other's viewpoints. Collaboration will be difficult if some members of the team feel the need to be in control, are critical of other team members, or are not able to share the responsibility.

The professional staff can contribute technical knowledge and experience with other children, but it is the parents who best understand their child and who must select the services that are best for that child. A true partnership between parents and professionals results in mutual respect, sharing of ideas, and ability to understand and learn from each other's viewpoints. Professionals need to be able to accept differences in family structures, culture, religious views, and other factors that affect daily living and child-rearing behaviors.

There are a variety of different structures for providing services. In some, the professional staff is in charge, make the majority of decisions, and the family is expected to follow the staff's recommendations. Depending on the specific program, the family will have different roles. In some, parents are expected to participate in educating the child; in others, the parents may have no role whatever in the child's therapy. In a more family-focused program, the parents select the program with the assistance of information provided by professionals. It is generally agreed that children will have the best opportunity for success if parents are intimately involved in all decisions and in treatment. In that way, they can follow up on treatment decisions at home and continue to provide appropriate language stimulation. The roles of all members of the team and their relative influence in program planning will change as the child moves from identification of a hearing loss, through extensive diagnosis, into education in preschool years, and into school years. Not every professional will be able to meet every family's needs. Some professionals feel more comfortable in a sign language environment and others prefer an oral–auditory environment. Not every child fits well into every program. Professionals need to recognize when they are not the appropriate person to be on a particular family's team and suggest that others substitute. As children develop, and as their program needs change, the team members may also need to change.

Diagnostic Evaluations

There are some basic evaluations that every child should have. Children with a serious case of otitis media may need different services than children with sensorineural hearing losses, but until the child has been evaluated, it will not be clear exactly what services are needed. Every child needs a pediatric evaluation, an otolaryngologic evaluation, a psychological/educational evaluation, and a speech-and-language evaluation. Children with sensorineural hearing loss also need an ophthalmologic evaluation. When any child is diagnosed with a sensorineural hearing loss of unknown origin, a genetics evaluation should be considered. After the basic evaluations, if there are other concerns, additional referrals will be requested. Evaluations can be provided by individual practitioners who do not work in the same facility but have a collaborative working arrangement. Some hospitals will have all the necessary specialists under one roof. Some community speech-and-hearing centers or educational programs will have therapeutic services in one facility but will frequently have to refer patients for medical evaluations. There are certainly advantages to having all services in one place. Professionals who work together regularly learn to communicate well with each other and can provide each other with assistance in making diagnoses. If parents select separate specialists who do not work in the same facility, one of the professionals should take responsibility for assisting parents in obtaining referrals and in collecting and understanding test results. This person may be the pediatrician who is managing the child's general health or, more frequently, is one of the specialists in hearing loss, usually the audiologist or otolaryngologist. (See the section, Team Manager, under Comprehensive Treatment Program, later in the chapter.)

The Basic Evaluations

Audiological Evaluations

The purpose of the initial audiological evaluation is to determine the degree and the type of hearing loss and to select amplification. Ongoing evaluations will monitor hearing; obtain additional information if the initial evaluation was not complete; monitor amplification; select new amplification, when needed; and monitor development of auditory functioning. Because the audiologist sees the infant or child on a more occasional basis (not daily or weekly, like parents, teachers, or therapists) she or he may be in a better position to monitor auditory functioning and development of auditory skills.

Pediatric Evaluation

The pediatric evaluation is necessary to monitor general health, to determine if there are any medical conditions, disorders, syndromes, or diseases (which may or may not be associated with hearing loss) that may have an affect on child development and to provide routine medical management.

Otolaryngological Evaluation

The goal of the otolaryngological evaluation is to examine the child for diseases of the head and neck, to determine whether the hearing loss is medically treatable, to identify the etiology of the hearing loss, and to determine if additional evaluations are indicated. The otolaryngologist may refer the child for blood tests, other medical tests, and radiological evaluations, if necessary, to assist in attempting to determine etiology of the hearing loss (Ruben, 1996; Madell, Gravel, & Ruben, 1995).

Genetics Evaluation

Any family with a child who has a hearing loss of unknown etiology should be referred for genetic counseling. Genetic counseling can provide two types of information: (a) assistance in determining the etiology of hearing loss, and (b) identification of associated medical conditions or syndromes that might need treatment. Some families choose not to seek genetic counseling, and that is their right; however, it is our responsibility to make the recommendation. This evaluation does not need to be scheduled immediately upon diagnosis, but can wait until the family is feeling more settled about the hearing loss and is prepared to move ahead.

Ophthamalogic Evaluation

Because a number of syndromes associated with hearing loss have ophthamalogic components, and because vision is critical to children with impaired hearing, all hearing-impaired children should be referred for ophthamalogic evaluation. Like genetics evaluations, this evaluation does not need to be scheduled immediately upon diagnosis but should be scheduled fairly early.

Psychological/Educational Evaluation

A psychological/educational evaluation provides important information about a child's development: It assists in identifying learning problems, provides information about which learning styles will be easiest and most difficult for the child, and determines if there are any additional developmental problems that may need to be addressed. One purpose of the psychological evaluation is to determine how the child compares with her or his normally hearing peers, and to monitor developmental progress over time. Selection of a psychologist to evaluate a hearing-impaired child is critical. Many psychological tests use language to determine intellectual and developmental level, which obviously is not appropriate for a hearing-impaired child. Using language as a measure of intellectual development can cause a hearing-impaired child to appear to have an intellectual delay that, in fact, she or he may not have. Using standardized tests on hearing-impaired children may also not be the best choice because the results cannot be easily compared with those of normally developing children and thus may give a skewed picture of the child's development. For assessing intellectual levels, nonverbal tests provide the best results, at least initially. A combination of verbal and nonverbal tests give a complete picture of the child's functioning.

Speech-and-Language Evaluation

A speech-and-language evaluation is essential for obtaining information about a child's receptive and expressive language skills, cognitive development, and ability to use audition. A speech pathologist who is experienced in working with hearing-impaired children and who has high expectations for the potential of hearing-impaired children should be selected for the evaluation. The information obtained from the speech-and-language evaluation will be of assistance in recommending educational placement.

Additional Evaluations

Neurological Evaluation

Any child for whom there is concern about physical, motor skills, or relational development, should be evaluated by a pediatric neurologist to determine if there are any disease or development processes that need identification and treatment. The pediatric neurologist will be able to identify disorders that may or may not be associated with hearing loss and can recommend medication; many pediatric neurologists who see multiply handicapped children with hearing loss can be helpful in discussing programs.

Occupational Therapy Evaluation

Children who have fine motor difficulties, balance difficulties, or difficulties with sensory issues (either hyper- or hyposensitivity to touch, taste, or vision) may benefit from occupational therapy. Some multiply handicapped hearing-impaired children need occupational therapy services.

Physical Therapy Evaluation

Physical therapy will be of assistance for children with gross motor problems, including difficulties with balance. Some multiply handicapped, hearing-impaired children need physical therapy services.

A Comprehensive Treatment Program

The staff of a child's treatment program may include the members of the diagnostic team or may have different practitioners from the same specialties. In either case, additional members will need to be added to the team. The primary team members are first and foremost, the parents, followed by the audiologist, the speech–language pathologist, the social worker, regular education teacher and/or special education teacher, otolaryngologist, pediatrician, and any other specialists that a particular child needs.

Funding

Funding is available through a variety of sources. Public Law 94–142 mandates appropriate educational services for all handicapped children in the least restrictive environment. The Individuals with Disabilities Education Act (IDEA), Part H, mandates early-intervention services for infants and toddlers and recognizes the role of the family in the provision of services. Services are determined through a team meeting, including parents, during which the Individual Family Service Plan (IFSP) is developed. The IFSP outlines the strengths and needs of the child and the family and the desired outcomes of intervention.

Although therapy services are frequently available, obtaining amplification is sometimes a problem. Some states, and some counties within states, provide hearing aids and frequency modulation (FM) systems to all children diagnosed with impaired hearing. In other states there is a financial means test, and in still other states, hearing aids are available but not FM systems. Individual health insurance may pay for hearing aids and therapy services if the hearing loss is the result of an accident or injury, but not if the hearing loss was present at birth. Some health insurance does not pay for speech-language therapy services, and others pay for only a limited number of visits.

Program Type

There are a variety of types of programs available. Different ones will be appropriate for different families. They range from full mainstreaming to schools for deaf children. Children who are fully mainstreamed may have no services (highly unusual) or may have any of the following: speech-language therapy, hearing therapy, resource room teacher, tutoring, notetakers, or in-class interpreters (oral, cued speech, American Sign Language or signed English.) Children may be partially mainstreamed, receiving some services in a regular classroom for some academic subjects or for social activities (e.g., gym, lunch), and receive other academic and tutorial services in a resource room or in a class for hearing-impaired, deaf, or language-impaired students. Some children will be in an inclusion program (a class with regular and special education students and teachers). Some children will be in a full-time classroom for hearing-impaired children in a regular school allowing them to receive academic work from a special education teacher but allowing for socialization with normally hearing children. Finally, some children will be enrolled in a school for the deaf in which all academic and special services are provided. Although children may be initially assigned to one program, they may move into other programs as they develop and their needs change. (Information about educational and communication options is available in Appendices 6, 7 and 8.)

Parents

The parents are, obviously, the most important members of the team. They need to indicate the direction for treatment and plan for services. The other team members are selected by the parents through suggestions from team members in the infant identification or treatment program, from other families, or from their own research. Most parents do not anticipate the birth of a hearing-impaired child and may initially have a difficult time putting together a team. This may require that the staff of the infant center to do the preliminary work until the family can take over.

Educational Management

When a child is identified with a handicapping condition, he or she is referred to the local agency responsible for evaluation and management. Programs differ from state to state. However, at the current time, most states have preschool evaluation teams and school-aged children are evaluated by evaluation teams located in their school district. The evaluation teams are usually comprised of members from a variety of different professions. Some teams will do all the evaluations and make recommendations for placement and the special services needed. Other teams obtain evaluations from professionals in the community and then meet to determine what services to recommend for a particular child. Many hearing-impaired children have no other diagnosis and need only a limited number of services. Others may have multiple problems and need a variety of therapies. The services that a child needs and the type of program the child is in will assist in determining who is a member of the team.

Team Manager

Every child needs a team manager (in addition to the parents). The team manager is responsible for being certain that the parents understand and agree with the recommendations, that all necessary services are being provided, that all team members are aware of what the other team members are doing, and that the child is re-evaluated on a regular basis to be certain that the program remains appropriate. If the children are not being seen within one building, it may be necessary to arrange team meetings on a regular basis so the team members can exchange observations and concerns. The team manager may change over time.

In an auditory–aural or auditory–visual treatment program the speech–language pathologist will frequently be the person who manages treatment, especially in the preschool years. Some audiologists are trained as auditory therapists and may take on this responsibility. Once the child reaches school age (nursery or elementary school), teachers become a critical part of the team. If the child is in a regular education program, the speech–language therapist may continue to be the team manager, or management may be the responsibility of the resource room teacher. The resource room teacher monitors classroom achievement, obtains work in advance, and may pre-teach material so that the child can function well in the mainstream classroom.

If the child is in a mainstreamed or inclusion setting, the therapists may be employed by the school and provide services within the school setting, or may be outside providers who provide services within the school setting or outside the school at their offices or at the child's home. In addition to providing speech–language services to the child, the speech–language pathologist assists the school staff in using amplification, in helping to explain hearing loss to other children, and in making the school staff feel comfortable with having a hearing-impaired child in the school.

If the child is in a special education setting, the responsibility for management will probably be shifted to the classroom teacher. All services will be provided in one setting and the classroom teacher is likely to be the person who is generally responsible for monitoring progress and recommending different services, when needed.

Auditory Management

The responsibilities of the audiologist are already well known. Because the audiologist is frequently the first person to discuss hearing loss with the family he or she is frequently the person who will provide a lot of the initial information and help the family get started. The audiologist will also continue to provide ongoing monitoring of hearing, amplification and auditory functioning, and determine when new amplification is needed. The audiologist needs to assist other members of the team in understanding how the amplification works, providing appropriate expectations for amplification, teaching school staff to use FM systems appropriately and to monitor hearing aids and FM systems. The audiologist is the appropriate person to make school visits to monitor amplification use, to assist the classroom teacher in maximizing the child's ability to hear all classroom discussion and in monitoring classroom noise. Some speech–language pathologists who work with hearing-impaired children will be able to perform the classroom monitoring if the audiologist is not a full-time member of the school team. However, if the speech pathologist is not comfortable doing this, the audiologist needs to make a visit.

Summary

Identification of hearing loss is only the first step in the management of a hearing-impaired child. Once the hearing loss has been identified, all other diagnostic evaluations need to be completed, educational/habilitation programs need to be selected, a program team needs to be developed and then the work begins. Each child and each family will have different needs and different teams will need to be developed. Collaborative efforts between team members and families will greatly enhance the final result—a well-adjusted, happy child and family with good communication skills.

References and Readings

Clark, K.A., & Terry, D.L. (1994). A collaborative framework for intervention. In Roeser, R., & Downs, M., (eds.): *Auditory Disorders in School Children.* New York: Thieme.

Hayes, D. & Northern, J. (1996). Components of an infant hearing program. In *Infants and Hearing.* San Diego: Singular Publishing.

Jung, J.H. (1989). *Genetic Syndromes in Communication Disorders.* Austin, TX: Pro-Ed.

Madell, J.R., Gravel, J., & Ruben, R.J. (1996). Otologic and Audiologic Evaluation: Hearing Loss in Infants. Paper presented at the 100th Annual Meeting, American Academy of Otolaryngology–Head and Neck Surgery Foundation, Inc., Washington, DC.

Marini, A., Read, A., & Stephens, D. (1996). *Genetics and Hearing Impairment.* San Diego: Singular Publishing.

Roush, J., & Matkin, N.D. (1994). *Infants and Toddlers with Hearing Loss: Family Centered Assessment and Intervention.* Baltimore: York Press.

Ruben, R.J. (1996). The Pediatric Otolaryngologic Assessment of the Child with a Suspected Hearing Loss. In Gerber, S. (ed.): *The Handbook of Pediatric Audiology.* Washington, DC: Gallaudet University Press.

APPENDIX 1

Joint Committee on Infant Hearing, 1994: Indicators Associated with Sensorineural and/or Conductive Hearing Loss

A. For use with neonates (birth through age 28 days) when universal screening is not available
   1) Family history of hereditary childhood sensorineural hearing loss
   2) In utero infection, such as cytomegalovirus, rubella, syphilis, herpes, or toxoplasmosis
   3) Craniofacial anomalies, including those with morphological abnormalities of the pinna and ear canal
   4) Birth weight less than 1500 g (3.3 lb)
   5) Hyperbilirubinemia at a serum level requiring exchange transfusion
   6) Ototoxic medications, including but not limited to the aminoglycosides, used in multiple courses or in combination with loop diuretics
   7) Bacterial meningitis
   8) Apgar scores of 0–4 at 1 minute or of 0–6 at 5 minutes
   9) Mechanical ventilation lasting 5 days or longer
   10) Stigmata or other findings associated with syndromes known to include a sensorineural and/or conductive hearing loss
B. For use with infants (age 29 days through 2 yr) when certain health conditions develop that require rescreening
   1) Parent/caregiver concern regarding hearing, speech, language, and/or developmental delay

2) Bacterial meningitis and other infections associated with sensorineural hearing loss

3) Head trauma associated with loss of consciousness or skull fracture

4) Stigmata or other findings associated with syndromes known to include a sensorineural and/or conductive hearing loss

5) Ototoxic medications, including but not limited to, chemotherapeutic agents or aminoglycosides, used in multiple courses or in combination with loop diuretics

6) Recurrent or persistent otitis media with effusion lasting at least 3 months

C. For use with infants and children (age 29 days through 3 yr) who require periodic monitoring of hearing

Some newborns and infants may pass initial hearing screening but require periodic monitoring of hearing to detect delayed-onset sensorineural and/or conductive hearing loss. Infants with these indicators require hearing evaluation at least every 6 months until the age of 3 years, and at appropriate intervals thereafter.

Indicators associated with delayed-onset sensorineural hearing loss include:

1) Family history of hereditary childhood hearing loss

2) In utero infection, such as cytomegalovirus, rubella, syphilis, herpes, or toxoplasmosis

3) Neurofibromatosis, type II, and neurodegenerative disorders.

Indicators associated with conductive hearing loss include:

1) Recurrent or persistent otitis media with effusion

2) Anatomic deformities and other disorders that affect eustachian tube function

3) Neurodegenerative disorders

APPENDIX 2

Case History Topics

1. Birth and Prenatal History
   Previous pregnancies
   Illnesses during the pregnancy, including week of pregnancy the illness
      occurred
   RH incompatibility, ABO blood incompatibility
   Medications, drugs (legal and illegal) taken during the pregnancy
   Complications during the pregnancy
   Length of the pregnancy
   Length of labor
   Delivery: cesarean section or vaginal
   Birth weight
   Complications at birth: anoxia, jaundice, Apgar scores, breech, other
   Length of hospitalization

2. Health History
   Colds
   Allergy
   Ear infections
   High fevers
   Immunizations
   Meningitis
   Other viruses (mumps, cytomegalovirus)
   Reactions to any of the above
   Immunization history, reaction to immunizations
   Drugs taken regularly

Drug reactions
Feeding or swallowing problems
Seizures

3. Developmental History
   Motor milestones: sitting, crawling, walking
   Age of visual response to parents
   Is walking clumsy? Does the child fall a lot?
   Feeding and eating history
   Age of toilet training

4. Communication History: Hearing
   What do parents think about the child's hearing?
   Sounds to which child responds
   Does she or he distinguish between sounds (phone, doorbell?)
   Does child want TV/radio loud?
   Does hearing fluctuate? Under what conditions?
   Are sounds uncomfortable? What sounds? Under what conditions?
   Amplification history: What amplification is/was used? Settings? Changes in amplification?

5. Communication History: Speech and Language
   Age of babbling, first word, phrases, sentences
   Does the child understand verbal requests with/without visual cues?
   How does the child communicate his or her needs? Voice, gesture, sign?
   Has there been a change in the child's speech and language? Did she or he speak and then stop?

6. Social History
   When did the child feed him or herself? Dress him or herself?
   Does she or he play with other children?
   What does the child like to play with?
   Does the child have any behavioral problems?
   How does the child get along with other children? Adults? Family members?
   Have there been any changes in the child's behavior?
   Does the child respond to others? Make eye contact?

7. Educational History
   Current school
   Type of educational program

Previous school placements
Special services received in school
Describe educational problems or concerns

8. Special Services
   What special services does the child receive in school? Outside of school?
   Speech–language therapy
   Hearing (auditory training) therapy
   Occupational therapy
   Physical therapy
   Psychological services
   Educational tutoring
   Other services

9. Other Evaluations
   What other evaluations has the child had (evaluator, dates, and results)?
   Audiological
   Speech–language
   Hearing (auditory training)
   Occupational therapy
   Physical therapy
   Psychological
   Educational
   Pediatric
   Otolaryngological
   Neurological
   Psychiatric
   Other evaluations

APPENDIX 3

Case History Form

IDENTIFYING INFORMATION Date_____

Name of Child_____ M_____ F_____ Date of birth_____
Address_____
_____ Zip code_____
Telephone_____ Referred by_____
Mother's full name_____Father's full name_____Guardian_____
Daytime phone _____ Daytime phone _____ Daytime phone _____
Medicaid #_____Medicare #_____ Private insurance_____
Parents' current status   Married_____ Divorced_____ Separated_____
Widowed_____ Single_____
Reason you are bringing this child for evaluation_____
_____
Has the child been referred to Early Intervention?_____ Committee on
Preschool Education?_____ Special education?_____
Others in home: (names, ages, and relationship)_____
_____
Have the other children ever had any of the following types of problems:
medical, academic, speech, hearing, emotional, or visual? _____ If so,
explain briefly_____
_____
Which languages are spoken at home?_____

What is the child's primary language?_____

Name of child's physician_____Address_____

BIRTH AND PRENATAL HISTORY

Mother's previous pregnancies (include miscarriages)_____

Any illnesses or complications during pregnancy with this child?_____

_____

List drugs/medication taken during this pregnancy_____

Length of pregnancy_____ Length of labor_____

Birth weight_____Was birth by Cesarian section?_____

Breech?_____ Did baby have anoxia (blue color) or respiratory

distress (breathing problems)?_____ jaundice (yellow color)_____

How long did the baby remain in the hospital?_____

COMPLICATIONS AT BIRTH

Scars, bruises, deformities?_____Difficulty sucking, swallowing, feed-

ing?_____

Other unusual conditions?_____

HEALTH HISTORY

Has the child had any of the following (give age/date)?_____

allergies_____asthma_____convulsions or seizures_____ear infections_____

frequent colds_____ high fever_____ swallowing problems_____

persistent sore throats_____ meningitis_____ mumps_____

rubella_____ sinus infections_____ blows to the head?_____exposure

to excessive noise?_____ Other_____ Are immunizations

up to date?_____ Reactions?_____ Has child ever been

hospitalized?_____ For what condition(s)?_____

_____

Has the child been tested for lead poisoning?_____ Has medication ever been used for control of convulsive disorders or emotional problems?_____

Does the child take any medications regularly?_____ If yes, which ones?_____

Has your child been seen by an eye doctor?_____ ear doctor?_____ neurologist?_____ psychologist?_____ If yes, give name, address, date and recommendations_____

_____

_____

List previous hearing tests and speech and language evaluations (place/date) _____

Has any member of your family had any of the following? What is the relationship to the child?

	Yes/No	Relationship
Deafness or hearing loss	_____	_____
Developmental delay	_____	_____
Language disorder	_____	_____
Speech/voice problem	_____	_____
Learning disability	_____	_____
Reading difficulty	_____	_____
Visual deficit	_____	_____
Psychological illness	_____	_____
Convulsive disorder	_____	_____
Other	_____	_____

DEVELOPMENTAL HISTORY

At what age did child: Show visual response to Mother_____ crawl_____ sit_____ Walk_____ Become toilet trained_____ Does your child have problems walking?_____ running?_____ climbing?_____ fall frequently?_____

At what age did child: babble?_____ imitate sounds?_____ say first word?_____ phrases?_____ sentences?_____

Does child understand verbal request, commands, directions, etc?_____

_____

How does child get what he or she wants? gesture_____ voice_____
voice and gesture_____ sign language_____ Describe a situation (i.e.,
"wanting bottle")_____

_____

Do you have concerns about your child's hearing?_____ Describe your
concerns_____
Does child respond to sounds when she or he can't see the source of the
sound?_____ If so, to what specific sounds_____
Does child want TV/radio excessively loud?_____ Does child distinguish
between different sounds? (e.g., phone vs doorbell, etc.)_____ Are there
sounds that make your child uncomfortable?_____
Does your child have tendency to "tune in and out" of listening situations?

_____

Does child wear a hearing aid?_____ FM system?_____ Who recommended
it?_____ When was it purchased?_____ When
does the child wear the hearing aid or FM? all the time_____ only at
school_____ in therapy_____ other_____
Name and model_____
Ear: right_____ left_____ both_____ Has child had any sudden changes in
hearing, speech, or behavior?_____ At what age did child begin to feed
him or herself?_____ Dress himself/herself?_____ Play with other
children?_____
Does he or she prefer playing alone?_____ List your child's favorite toys
or games_____
Is your child's behavior easily managed at home?_____ at school?_____
How does your child get along with other members of the family?_____

_____

_____

Has this child's development been in any way different from that of the
other children in your family? (If your answer is yes, please describe)_____

_____

_____

SCHOOL INFORMATION

What school does your child attend?_____Grade_____

Address_____ Phone_____ Principal_____

Classroom Teacher_____List previous schools and dates attended

_____

If child has received special services at school (resource room, remedial reading, speech therapy, supplemental help, bilingual class, special class or school, psychological evaluation, etc.) please answer the following section.

Type of Service   How Often?   Date Received   Name of Specialist

_____   _____   _____   _____

_____   _____   _____   _____

_____   _____   _____   _____

If child has received special services privately (evaluation and/or treatment: psychological, psychiatric, neurological, speech, hearing visual, educational, medical, other) please answer the following:

Type of Service   How Often?   Date Received   Name of Specialist

_____   _____   _____   _____

_____   _____   _____   _____

_____   _____   _____   _____

Do you have any questions you want answered by this evaluation?

Completed by_____

Relationship to child_____

APPENDIX 4

Simple Case History Form

Questions at 3 months

Yes	No		Yes	No	
—	—	1. Jumps (startles at sudden loud sounds)	—	—	1. Has a special cry when hungry
—	—	2. Stirs from sleep when there is a loud noise	—	—	2. Coos when fed and dry
—	—	3. Stops sucking when there is a sudden new sound	—	—	3. Laughs
—	—	4. Smiles at mother	—	—	4. Holds head up staight while lying on the stomach

Questions at 6 months

Yes	No		Yes	No	
—	—	1. Turns in the general direction of a new or sudden sound	—	—	1. Seems to enjoy making sounds with voice, like "baba", "ooh, ooh"
—	—	2. Usually stops crying when mother talks to baby	—	—	2. Chuckles, gurgles, or laughs when playing
—	—	3. Enjoys a musical toy	—	—	3. Makes happy sound when sees s/he is going to be fed
—	—	4. Reaches out to be picked up by someone in the family	—	—	4. Rolls over, either from back to front or from front to back

Questions at 9 months

Yes	No		Yes	No	
__	__	1. Responds to his or her name, to "no" and "bye-bye"	__	__	1. Imitates speech but doesn't use real words
__	__	2. Knows if a person's voice sounds friendly or angry	__	__	2. Seems to be using "own words" to name things
__	__	3. Looks directly at a new sound or voice	__	__	3. Makes a lot more and different sounds than a couple of months ago
__	__	4. Plays peek-a-boo	__	__	4. Sits well without any help

From Matkin, N. (1984). Early recognition and referral of hearing-impaired children. *Pediatr in Rev, 6*, 153. Adapted with permission.

APPENDIX 5

Familiar Sounds Audiogram

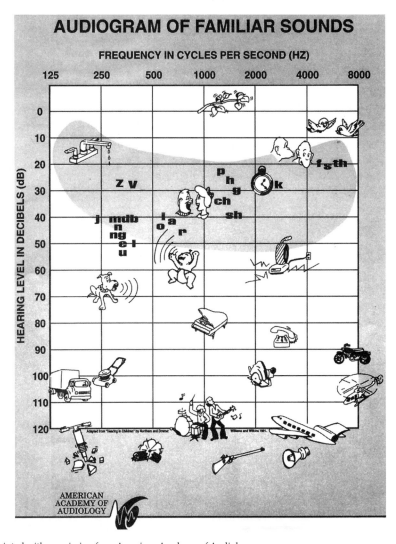

Reprinted with permission from American Academy of Audiology.

APPENDIX 6

Basic Information for Parents about Hearing Loss

What is a Hearing Loss?

A hearing loss is the reduced ability to hear sound. There are many different types and degrees of hearing loss. Hearing loss varies from mild to profound. It may occur in one or both ears, and may be present at birth or develop later.

What Causes Hearing Loss in Children?

Hearing loss can be caused by illnesses the mother had during pregnancy or difficulties during the birth. Some childhood illnesses, such as rubella, mumps, certain viruses, meningitis, and high fevers, cause hearing loss. Exposure to certain drugs or medications has also been known to cause hearing loss. Many childhood hearing losses are thought to be caused by hereditary factors; some are dominant (the gene is carried by only one parent) and others are recessive (the gene is carried by both parents.) Hereditary hearing losses can occur when there is no known hearing loss in the family. Hearing losses that are present at birth are called congenital. Hearing losses that develop after birth are called acquired. Colds and ear infections can cause hearing loss but the loss is usually temporary.

How Does the Ear Work?

The ear has several parts. The part you see on the side of the head is called the pinna. It catches sound and passes it down the ear canal toward the eardrum. The pinna and the ear canal are called the outer ear. On the other side of the eardrum is the middle ear. It contains the 3 small bones that carry the sound waves from the eardrum into the inner ear, two "windows" between the middle and inner ear covered by membranes, and the eustachian tube, which runs from the middle ear into the throat. The inner ear consists of the cochlear, which is a snail shell-shaped bone containing the hair cells that respond to the sound transmitted from the bones in the middle ear. The hair cells transmit sound to the auditory nerve, which carries the sound to the brain, where it is interpreted. The inner ear also contain the semicircular canals that control balance.

Are There Different Types of Hearing Losses?

There are two types of hearing loss. Conductive hearing loss is caused by damage to the outer or middle ear. Sensorineural hearing loss is caused by damage to the inner ear. A mixed hearing loss is a combination of conductive and sensorineural hearing loss.

How is Hearing Loss Treated?

Hearing loss caused by colds or ear infections frequently clears up on its own. If it does not, it is usually easily treated with medication or, in some cases, with pressure-equalization tubes that allow fluid to drain from the middle ear into the ear canal. Some children are born with physical deformities of the outer or middle ear, which can sometimes be corrected through surgery. Children with this type of deformity also do very well with hearing aids. Sensorineural or inner ear hearing loss cannot be corrected surgically. Children with sensorineural hearing losses do well with hearing aids and with therapy to assist in learning language.

Do Hearing Aids Help?

Hearing aids are not perfect but, fortunately, they help a great deal. Hearing aids are not like eyeglasses. They do not help immediately. You child will need to learn to use hearing aids and will need to learn to listen to sound and speech. When children wear hearing aids for the first time, they have to go through all the learning stages that normal hearing children go through before they learn to talk or to understand their parents. This takes time. There are many different kinds of hearing aids, and your audiologist will assist you in selecting the best hearing aids for your child and in helping you and your child learn to use them. Almost every child benefits from two hearing aids. We do better with two ears in the same way that we do better with two eyes. There is research indicating that people who do not wear hearing aids may lose some of their ability to use their hearing in the unaided ear. Some children who do not receive enough help from hearing aids may benefit from a cochlear implant, a hearing aid that is implanted into the cochlear and is attached by a magnet to a small wearable computer. Please be patient and continue to talk, talk, talk to your hearing-impaired child so she or he can learn to use hearing and hearing aids.

How Early Should We Begin?

Identification and treatment should begin as early as possible because hearing loss affects a child's speech, language, and academic learning. As soon as parents become concerned about their child's hearing, the child should have a hearing evaluation by an audiologist. **NO CHILD IS EVER TOO YOUNG TO TEST.** The audiologist will be able to determine if the child has a hearing loss, and how much and what type of a hearing loss the child has. The child should also be evaluated by an otolaryngologist (a physician who specializes in diseases of the ear). The otolaryngologist will determine if the hearing loss can be treated medically, and if other medical tests or evaluations are needed. After the hearing loss has been diagnosed by the audiologist and otolaryngologist, habilitation (treatment) can begin. The first step is getting the right hearing aids. Next, parents need to select the type of therapy program that they wish for their child and arrange for therapy to assist them and the child in learning to communicate. Hearing loss affects learning language, so it is very important that treatment begin as early as possible. A variety of therapy programs is available. The audiologist will assist families in learning about different kinds of therapy programs and locating one that works well for them. Children need to listen for a long time before they can learn to talk or to understand speech. Be patient and **TALK, TALK, TALK** to your child.

When you have questions, contact your audiologist, otolaryngologist, speech–language pathologist, or hearing education teacher. They are all available to help you.

APPENDIX 7

Amplification Options for Children with Impaired Hearing

Ninety-five percent of children who have hearing losses have some residual hearing (hearing they can learn to use). Making optimal use of a child's residual hearing is greatly to his or her benefit. Learning to use residual hearing requires: (a) the correct amplification system, and (b) a therapy program to help children learn to use hearing to their maximal ability. It is very important that children have the best possible hearing aids with the best possible sound quality because they will be using hearing aids to learn speech and language, to learn in school, and to communicate with the world.

What Kinds of Amplification Systems Are There?

There are several different kinds of amplification systems: hearing aids, FM systems, tactile aids, and cochlear implants.

Hearing Aids

Hearing aids come in different sizes and different strengths and are specifically selected for each child by an audiologist, who takes into account the child's hearing loss, age, size, and listening needs. They are worn individually on each ear. Hearing aids amplify all sound, speech as well as noise. All hearing aids work best when the child is within 3 to 6 feet of the person who is speaking and when there is no background noise.

BEHIND-THE-EAR HEARING AIDS

Behind-the-ear hearing aids are the most common hearing aids for young children. They are shaped like a half-moon, are worn behind the child's ear, and are attached to the ear by an earmold (a piece of molded plastic that is shaped to fit the individual's ear). Behind-the-ear hearing aids come in different strengths and can be adjusted to help different hearing losses. The adjustments can be changed as more is learned about the child's hearing or if hearing changes. The advantage to behind-the-ear hearing aids is that they can be adjusted to meet the child's changing needs.

BODY-WORN HEARING AIDS

Body-worn hearing aids have all components encased in a small box, usually worn in a pocket, and are attached to the ear by a cord that connects the body aid to an earmold (a piece of molded plastic that is shaped to fit the individual's ear). Body-worn hearing aids are used less frequently than other types of hearing aids and primarily for situations in which in-the-ear or behind-the-ear hearing aids do not work well. For very young children who cannot sit up, a body-worn hearing aid may be easier to use. It may also be more powerful. Because the microphone is several inches away from the earmold, there is less feedback.

TRANSPOSER HEARING AID

A transposer hearing aid is a special kind of body-worn hearing aid used for children and adults who have profound hearing losses and do not benefit from standard hearing aids. Some people with profound hearing losses hear sound in the low pitches but not in the high pitches. The transposer hearing aid transposes the sounds that occur in the high pitches and put them into the low pitches where the person has better hearing. Sound from this kind of hearing aid would seem strange to a person with normal hearing but works well for people with certain kinds of hearing losses.

IN-THE-EAR AND IN-THE-CANAL HEARING AIDS

In-the-ear and in-the-canal hearing aids are molded to the person's ear and fit entirely in the outer ear and in the ear canal. They are popular because they are small and less visible. These hearing aids must fit perfectly to work well. They are not good for young children for several reasons: their ears are usually too small to fit all the parts and, because their ears grow quickly, the hearing aid needs be remade often. This can occur more than once a year and can be very expensive. It can be difficult to make these hearing aids powerful enough for severe and profound hearing losses.

FM Systems

FM systems were designed to solve some of the problems that hearing aids do not solve, such as listening at more than 3 feet and listening in noise. Hearing aids work best when the child is within 3 to 6 feet of the person who is speaking and when there is no background noise. If the talker is more than a few feet away, the child will hear the talker plus all the noise in between. For example, if the room is noisy, if a television or radio is on, if there are other people talking, or if children are playing with toys, it will be very hard for the child to hear clearly. Although everyone has some difficulty hearing in noisy places, people who have hearing losses have much more difficulty. This is a very serious problem in a classroom, but it can also be a problem at home, especially for young children with severe and profound hearing losses.

FM systems have two parts: a receiver, worn by the hearing-impaired person, and a microphone, worn by the talker. The signal is sent from the microphone to the receiver by FM radio waves. There are several different kinds of FM systems. Some have hearing aids built into them so that you do not need separate hearing aids, and some are attached to hearing aids. Some fit behind the ear and some are worn in a box like a body hearing aid. The choice of a specific FM system depends on the individual's needs.

Every child with any degree of hearing loss will need an FM system for school because schools are very noisy places. An FM system is also useful in noisy situations at home, such as at the dinner table, while watching TV, or while riding in the car. Some children, especially those with severe and profound hearing losses, will benefit from wearing an FM system full time at home.

BEHIND-THE-EAR FM SYSTEM

A behind-the-ear FM system is built into a behind-the-ear hearing aid. It can be used as a hearing aid, without FM, as an FM system without a hearing aid, or as both an FM system and a hearing aid at the same time. It can be adapted to almost all degrees of hearing loss.

BODY-WORN FM

A body-worn FM system is worn in a pocket, like a body-worn hearing aid. It has the advantage of being sturdy and easily adjustable, depending on the child's hearing loss. There is an additional advantage for very young children: A body-worn FM system can help reduce feedback (that whistling sound). It is frequently very difficult for young children (especially those with severe and profound hearing losses) to wear hearing aids without the hearing aids producing feedback. Feedback is caused by an air leak between the hearing aid microphone, the earmold, and the ear. Part of the problem is that a young child's ear is very soft, which contributes to an air leak. A body-worn FM helps reduce feedback because the microphone is on the box several inches away from the child's ear and therefore, the earmold fit doesn't have to be so tight.

Tactile Aids

Tactile aids are used for children who have profound hearing loss and who do not benefit from standard hearing aids. Tactile aids use a vibrator that is placed on the wrist, the collar bone, or the stomach. As a person talks, the signal is sent through the vibrator and the child receives the rhythm of speech. It is very difficult to understand speech using a tactile aid alone, but tactile aids can be helpful in combination with speechreading.

Cochlear Implants

Cochlear implants are very powerful hearing aids that are implanted in the inner ear. They are recommended for people who have not benefited from standard hearing aids. Surgery is required to implant the electrodes into the inner ear. A small magnet is placed under the scalp to connect the internal part to a small computer, which is worn on a belt or in a pocket. The computer is programmed for the individual person's hearing.

Does Everyone who has a Hearing Loss Need Hearing Aids?

If a hearing loss is mild, a hearing-impaired person may hear well in a variety of situations but will have difficulty hearing when it is noisy or when the person speaking is more than 6 feet away. Adults may be able to manage, but children will have difficulty because they are learning language and academics. Almost everyone with a hearing loss has difficulty hearing in some situations. If those situations are important (such as school), hearing aids are also important.

Do You Always Need Two Hearing Aids?

Research has demonstrated that an ear that is not used will lose the ability to understand speech. Therefore, hearing aids should be worn on both ears if there is a hearing loss in both ears. We would not consider wearing eyeglasses on only one eye!

How Is the Right Amplification System Selected?

An audiologist selects an amplification system based on expert technical knowledge and experience with other children with similar hearing losses and then evaluates how the system works on the child. The testing is similar to that done without hearing aids and will be compared with the unaided testing and with normal hearing to find a system that provides good benefit. After the child has been wearing the hearing aid or FM system for a few weeks she or he will be retested to determine if it is still providing the expected benefit or needs to be adjusted. Amplification systems for children need to be checked several times a year.

How Can I Be Sure My Child Is Getting the Most from Hearing Aids?

Unfortunately, hearing aids are not like eyeglasses. You don't just put them on and solve the hearing problem the way eyeglasses solve vision problems. Children need to be taught to use the residual hearing that is made available to them with their hearing aids. They need to be carefully taught to listen and to understand speech using hearing. This is best done with the help of an audiologist or speech–language therapist who can work with the child and help teach him or her the necessary skills. They also need to be taught how to take care of their hearing aids so that, if the battery dies or the hearing aid falls out when a parent is not around, they can fix the problem themselves. These are their "ears" and they must learn to care for them.

How Often Do Hearing Aids Need to be Fixed or Replaced?

Hearing aids usually last between 3 to 5 years. They need to be checked very carefully several times a year to be certain they are working well because they may break down and need repair. It is especially important that children's hearing aids be checked frequently because children use the hearing aids to learn language and to learn in school.
DISCUSS ALL QUESTIONS ABOUT HEARING AIDS AND FM SYSTEMS WITH YOUR AUDIOLOGIST.

APPENDIX 8

Educational Options for Children with Impaired Hearing

There are a variety of options available for educating hearing-impaired infants and children. The decision about how to select the best program for a particular child and his or her family is usually overwhelming because parents are asked to make these important decisions at a time when they have just learned that they have a child who is hearing impaired and may know very little about hearing loss.

What are the Educational Options for Educating Children who Have Impaired Hearing?

There are four different types of educational programs for educating children who are hearing impaired: total communication, auditory–oral, auditory–verbal and cued-speech programs. Not every child will do well in every program. Selection of a particular program for a particular child depends on many things, including the child's age at the time of diagnosis, other problems the child may have unrelated to hearing loss, the family's ability to help teach the child, and the quality of the specific programs where the family lives.

Total Communication

Total communication uses a combination of sign language and speech. Children wear hearing aids, but most total communication programs emphasize sign language rather than listening as part of therapy. The advantage of total communication is that children can learn language quickly since signs are readily visible and easy to understand. Parents and others who interact with the child *must* learn to sign or they will not be able to communicate with the child and will not be able to help the child learn.

The idea of teaching children to speak and to sign at the same time is a good one, and although most children who are educated in total communication programs develop good sign language skills, many do not develop good speech skills. This occurs for several reasons. First, because the adults are signing and speaking at the same time, the children pay attention to the signs that are easier for them to understand and do not attend as well to the speech or sound, which is more difficult to understand. In addition, American Sign Language (ASL) uses a different grammar than speech, making it difficult to follow both ASL and speech at the same time. (It is like listening to two different languages at the same time.) The reading level of high school graduates educated in total communication programs is about 5th grade. Part of the reason for this is that the grammar used in everyday conversation is different from that of written language. There are some programs that use signed English, which is a different language than ASL, and uses the same grammar as standard English. However, this system is not used by the deaf community so it does not allow the child to speak with other deaf people.

People who favor total communication feel that sign language allows the deaf child to be a member of the deaf community and to communicate easily within that group. They are concerned that children who do not learn sign will not learn to communicate and will be isolated. Although socialization with the deaf community is much easier in sign, socialization and work with people who do not sign is more difficult.

Children who are educated in total communication programs attend schools for the deaf or special classes in public schools where the teachers and other students sign.

Auditory–Oral Education

The goal of an auditory–oral program is to teach a child to speak, and to learn to understand the speech of others through speechreading or lipreading (watching a person's face) and through listening with hearing aids. All children wear hearing aids. The advantage to an auditory–oral education is that children who learn to speak will be able to talk to everyone because they are speaking the same language. Not every child can successfully learn to speechread. Speechreading can be difficult because some sounds (such as *p*, *b*, and *m*) look the same on the lips. For this reason, speechreading needs to be combined with using hearing aids to help the child understand. This kind of program requires a great deal of effort on the part of the family for the child to be successful. Children who are educated in an auditory–oral education program have the option of being mainstreamed (going to school with children who are not hearing-impaired) or educated in special classes with other hearing-impaired children either in public schools or in special schools. If the children are in mainstreamed classes, they will probably receive special assistance from a teacher of hearing-impaired children to assist with academic tutoring, and from a speech–language pathologist who will assist with speech and language skills.

Auditory–Verbal Education

Auditory-verbal therapy is an extension of auditory-oral therapy. The auditory–verbal philosophy is that almost all hearing-impaired children can learn to use the hearing they have with appropriate hearing aids. The hearing-impaired child is taught to rely on residual hearing to learn language and to monitor his or her speech. Sign language is not used and speechreading is discouraged, at least when learning new language. The right hearing aid or FM system is critical to this method because learning relies on using residual hearing. Not every child can successfully learn to use residual hearing. Children who are educated in an auditory–verbal education program have the option of being mainstreamed (going to school with children who are not hearing impaired); they may be educated in special classes with other hearing impaired children in their public schools or in special schools. If the children are in mainstreamed classes, they will probably receive special assistance from a teacher of hearing-impaired children to assist with academic tutoring, and from a speech–language pathologist who will assist with speech and language skills and continue to improve their auditory skills.

Cued Speech

Cued speech is an oral method. Children rely on speechreading and hand signals, which help distinguish among the speech sounds that look alike on the lips. For example, p and b, which look the same on the lips, have different hand cues to help distinguish them. Cues are not signs and cannot be understood by themselves. They are useful only when combined with speechreading. It is hoped that children will learn language with cued speech and then drop the cues and rely on speechreading. Some children go to school with a cued-speech interpreter to assist in receiving information.

How Can I Decide Which Program Is Best for My Child and Our Family?

Programming decisions are very difficult and can only be made after a great deal of thought. Before making a placement decision for your child, you should visit the programs and individual therapists in your community, talk to the parents of other hearing-impaired children who are enrolled in different programs, and talk to older hearing-impaired teens and adults who have been educated in different kinds of programs.

What if I Make the Wrong Decision?

Every programming decision should be reviewed on a regular basis. Not every program is right for every child. As the child grows and learns, you and the therapists will know more about what is best. At the beginning, the child's progress should be reviewed several times a year. If the program you have chosen is not right, or if your child is not progressing as originally expected, a change can be considered.

ADDITIONAL INFORMATION

1. Auditory–Verbal International
2121 Eisenhower Avenue,
Suite 402
Alexandria, VA
703–739–1049

2. The Alexander Graham Bell
Association for the Deaf
3417 Volta Place, NW
Washington, DC 20007–2778
202–337–5220
(for auditory oral and auditory verbal information)

3. Cued Speech National Center
P.O. Box 31345
Raleigh, NC 27622–1345
919–828–1218

4. National Information Center for
the Deaf
Gallaudet University
800 Florida Avenue, NE
Washington, DC 20002
202–651–5051
(for sign language and total communication)

APPENDIX 9

Checking Amplification Systems

The hearing aids or FM system that your child wears are his or her ears. It is very important that they work well. You must check them every day to be certain that they are working, especially because young children will not be able to report problems. In the beginning it may be difficult for you to tell if the system is working well, but after testing it daily for a while, you will be able to tell if it is working well. If something is wrong, try to solve the problems with the suggestions listed below. If you cannot solve the problem, bring the system back to your audiologist or hearing aid dispenser for help.

Equipment Needed for Checking Amplification Systems

1. Earmold or listening tube
2. Battery tester
3. Earmold blower for cleaning the earmold
4. Extra batteries, cords, audio-input boots, etc.
   Keep all supplies in a box or bag so they can be easily located.

Daily Listening Check

1. Visually inspect the system. Are earmolds clean and free of debris, and not clogged with earwax? Check that the microphone openings are clear and that all the settings are correct. Check the case to be certain it is not cracked and that it is free of debris and dirt. If the system has cords, check that they are not frayed.

2. Using an earmold or listening tube, listen to the system. Talk in sentences so you can hear what speech sounds like. Then say some speech sounds (*aaa, eee, uuuu, mmmm, shshshsh, sssss*) and listen to be certain they are heard clearly. If you are listening to a powerful system, squeeze the listening tube to reduce the sound reaching your ear. This will make it more comfortable to listen to and protect your hearing.

3. While listening, wiggle cords, hearing aid, volume control, switches, and connectors to be certain that there are no short-circuits or loose connections.

4. Check each hearing aid separately. If your child is wearing a body-worn FM system, be certain to check each side separately. With a body-worn or behind-the-ear FM system, check each hearing aid separately with and without the FM turned on. (With an FM system you will need to check 4 times: each hearing aid alone and each hearing aid with FM.)

Electronic Checking of Amplification

Children should have their amplification systems checked by the audiologist or the hearing aid dispenser several times a year. This will identify any distortion in the system or any other problems that require that the system be returned to the manufacturer for repair.

Cleaning the System

1. Earmolds get dirty and clogged with wax. To clean, remove them from the hearing aid, and wash with warm water and mild soap. Use the earmold blower to blow out any water left in the mold before reattaching it to the hearing aid. Clean earmolds at night so they have several hours to dry out before being reattached to the hearing aid.

2. Clean the case, using a clean moist cloth. Do not get any moisture into the hearing aid. Turn all dials and switches to loosen any dirt or debris.

Hearing Aid Troubleshooting Guide

When diagnosing a problem, to follow these steps:
1. Turn the system off, then on, to reset the system.
2. Ensure that the fitter controls are set correctly.

	No Sound	*Intermittent or Static*	*Weak or Distorted*	*Feedback*
Recharge or replace batteries	•	•	•	
Check cords/ tubing	•	•	•	
Check transducer	•	•	•	•
Check fitter controls	•	•	•	•
Turn up volume	•		•	
Clean or replace earmolds	•		•	•

FM Troubleshooting Guide

When diagnosing a problem, follow these steps:
1. If another working system is available, interchange accessories to locate the problem.
2. Turn the system off, then on, to reset the system.
3. Ensure the fitter controls are set correctly.

	No Sound	No FM	Intermittent or Static	Weak or Distorted	Feedback	Won't Charge
Recharge or replace batteries	•	•	•	•		•
Check cords/tubing	•	•	•	•		
Check transducer	•		•	•	•	
Check boot/shoe	•	•	•			
Check headset	•		•	•		
Check fitter controls	•	•	•	•	•	
Check that channels match	•	•	•	•		
Turn up volume	•	•		•		
Check microphone	•	•	•			
Clean or replace earmold	•			•	•	
Check hearing aid tubing					•	
Check charger						•
Clean charge contacts						•

APPENDIX 10

Using an FM System

What Is an FM System?

With a standard hearing aid, a hearing-impaired child will hear well if she or he is close to the person who is speaking and if there is no background noise. The farther away the talker is from the listener and the more noisy the setting is, the more problems the hearing-impaired child will have listening. With a mild hearing loss, the problems of noise and distance may be minimal, but as the hearing loss becomes more severe, listening will be more difficult. The FM system is a listening system designed to overcome the negative effects of distance and competing noise. It has 2 parts, a receiver worn by the hearing impaired child and a microphone/transmitter worn by the person who is speaking. The microphone transmits speech over FM radio waves to the receiver. The receiver may have a hearing aid in it in addition to the FM receiver, in which case the child will not need additional hearing aids, or the FM receiver may be attached to the child's hearing aids with wires or a teleloop.

The FM Transmitter

The real advantage of an FM system, compared with standard hearing aids, is the use of the transmitter. The transmitter is an extra microphone that is used by a parent, teacher, friend or therapist that enables the hearing-impaired child to hear what the other person is saying as if the speaker were talking directly into the microphone on the child's hearing aid. No matter how far away the speaker is from the hearing-impaired child, or how much noise there is between the hearing-impaired child and the person speaking, the sound will come in clearly. (How much of the sound the person hears and understands will depend on the hearing loss and the ability to use residual hearing, but by using and FM system, it is certain that a clear signal is being received.)

The FM Receiver

There are several different kinds of FM receivers. Some have hearing aids in them, and some are only receivers. The ones that have hearing aids may be in a case that looks like a behind-the-ear hearing aid (Figure 10A–1) or may be in a case like a body worn hearing aid (Figure 10A–2). These systems come in different strengths and have settings that need to be adjusted by the audiologist, depending on the child's hearing loss. If a body-worn system is being used with button transducers, it should be worn outside the child's clothing and about 6 inches below his or her mouth so that she or he can hear herself or himself talk and not get interference from clothing rubbing on the system. Some children wear their own behind the ear hearing aids and plug the FM receiver into the hearing aid (direct audio input) (Figure 10A–3). Others use their own hearing aids, switch them to the "telephone" setting and use the telephone coil of the hearing aid to pick up a signal from a magnetic loop worn in a wire around the neck (Figure 10A–4). An audiolo-

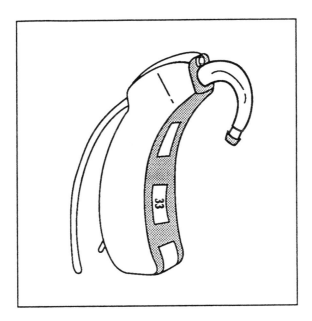

Figure 10A–1.   Behind-the-ear hearing aid/FM system. (Courtesy of Phonic Ear, Inc.)

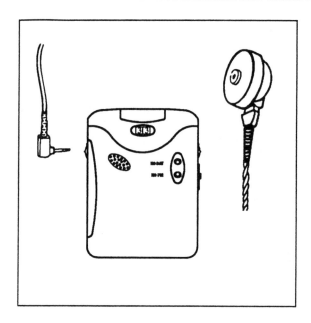

Figure 10A–2.   Body worn hearing aid/FM system. (Courtesy of Phonic Ear, Inc.)

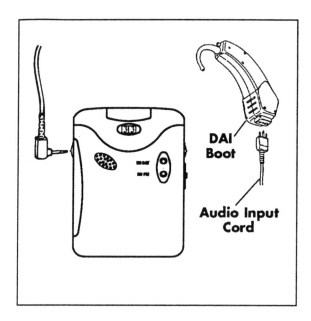

Figure 10A–3.   FM system with direct audio input to BTE hearing aid. (Courtesy of Phonic Ear, Inc.)

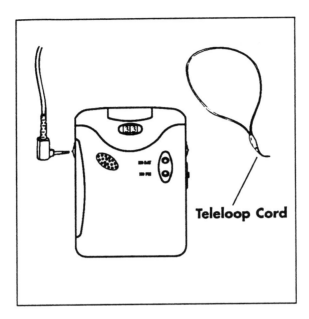

Teleloop Cord

Figure 10A–4. FM system with neck loop. (Courtesy of Phonic Ear, Inc.)

gist will help determine which system is most appropriate for each individual.

How to Wear the FM System

If the FM receiver is being worn with hearing aids or behind-the-ear transducers, the receiver can be worn in a pocket or attached to a belt. If button receivers are being used, with a body-worn FM, the unit should be worn on the chest with the microphones located 6 to 8 inches from the user's mouth so that he or she can hear his or her own voice clearly, as well as the voices of those standing close by. The receiver can be worn under clothing, but this will add noise from the clothing rubbing on the microphones and can muffle the sound, so it should be avoided. For young children, it is best to use a pocket or harness that has a loose cover over the top to keep food and dirt from falling into the microphone's openings and damaging the FM.

Using the Transmitter

The purpose of the transmitter (Figure 10A–5) is to send a clear signal from the person who is speaking to the listener. The transmitter should be placed

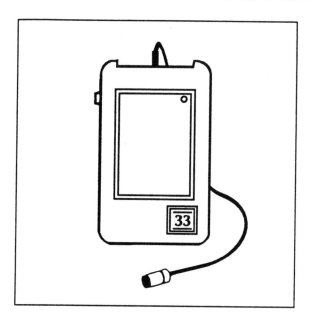

Figure 10A–5. FM transmitter. (Courtesy of Phonic Ear, Inc.)

6 to 8 inches from the speaker's mouth and should not be covered by clothing to ensure that a clear signal is being transmitted. It is not necessary to use the transmitter if the speaker and the hearing-impaired listener are sitting close together because the listener can hear through the microphones on her or his hearing aids. The transmitter should not be used if the speaker is in a different room and having a conversation that does not involve the hearing-impaired child. Using the transmitter in that situation will only be confusing and will interfere with the meaningful sound coming into the microphone on the hearing-impaired child's unit. If the child's FM is on and you do not want him or her to hear you, turn the transmitter to the AUX position. The child will hear through her or his hearing aids, but not through the microphone. Do not turn the microphone "off" or the child will hear interference. The transmitter microphone should be turned on when the speaker wants to talk to the hearing-impaired listener and turned off when communicating with someone else.

FM systems transmit signals on one of more than 30 different frequencies. Some FM systems use narrow-band channels, which transmit using a narrow-band signal. Others transmit using a wide-band signal made up of several narrow-band channels. It is important to check to see that both the transmitter and receiver frequencies match. If more than one FM system is being used in the same place (like a classroom) both children should be using the same channel. If two FM systems are being used but they are being used by two different listeners and speakers, the systems should be set on different frequencies or the children may have interference. Interference can also be received from fluorescent lights and from other radio signals. If interference is a problem, try a different channel.

The FM transmitter should be used any time the parent, teacher, therapist or play partner is more than a few feet from the child, or when there is competing noise. This will ensure that the child is receiving a clear sound and will facilitate learning language and academic materials.

APPENDIX 11

A Letter to the Classroom Teacher

Dear Teacher,

I am writing on behalf of J., who is a patient of mine and a student of yours. I am certain that we both have his or her best interests at heart, and I am writing to you for assistance in providing him or her with all the help that he or she needs to be the excellent student that he or she has the potential to be.

J. has a moderately severe sensorineural hearing loss in both ears. This means that without hearing aids, she or he will hear people when they are talking in a louder-than-normal voice standing near her or him. With hearing aids, J. will hear well if there is no noise and if he or she is close (within 3 to 4 ft) to the person who is talking. If the room is noisy (like any classroom filled with children, even if they are very well behaved) or if the person talking is more than a few feet away, J. will not hear as well. Even under the best of conditions, a person who has a hearing loss does not hear things as clearly as someone with normal hearing. It is like listening to a radio that is not quite on the station. Sometimes a person with a hearing loss can manage even without hearing everything by guessing from the things that he or she can hear. However, this causes a great deal of strain. It is a lot of work to have to concentrate constantly and guess at what is being said. Although it is possible to do this for a short time, it is not easy to do for an entire day. The more important the learning is, the more important it is that every word be heard, and the more strain is caused by the effort.

Preferential Seating

There are two things that can be done to help J. hear well in the classroom and learn well in school: preferential seating in the front of the room and use of an FM listening system.

J. must be seated in the front of the room to be able both to see and to hear the teacher and to be closer to the important source of speech. However, even when sitting in the front of the room it will not be possible to hear everything that is said because even the best behaved children make noise. The seats squeak, shoes make noise on the floor, papers rustle, children cough, etc. and these noises will interfere with the ability to hear the teacher even when the teacher is close by.

Using an FM System

The best way to improve J.'s listening is with an FM system, which is a listening system in which the teacher wears a microphone and the child wears a radio receiver. For the system to work well, the microphone must be within 6 inches of the mouth of the person who is speaking. If it is farther away, the microphone will pick up the other noises in the classroom and they will be amplified along with the teacher's speech. If J. is to do his best in school and not be under any unnecessary strain, it is essential that the teacher's voice be as clear as possible. This means that the FM system must be used all the time and must be worn at the correct distance from the mouth of the person who is speaking.

There will be times when you are talking to other children privately, or to another teacher, and when it is not necessary for J. to hear what you are saying—when, in fact, it might interfere with something else that he is doing. When this is the case, simply turn the FM transmitter that you are wearing to the AUX position. Do not turn it off if J.'s FM is still on. If you turn it off, J.'s FM may emit interference, which is very unpleasant to listen to. If you have it turned to the AUX position, J. will still be able to hear from her or his hearing aids, but will not hear you. When you are ready to talk to J. again, simply turn the transmitter back to MIC and he will hear you.

Facilitating Classroom Listening and Learning

As I have said, a classroom is a noisy place. Although hearing aids and FMs help, they do not solve all of the problems. Hearing aids will help J. hear speech that is close by, and the FM will help for speech within a few inches of the microphone. When other children are speaking, it will be difficult for a child with a hearing loss to hear. It is important for academic reasons that J. hear what is going on in classroom discussion and it is important for social reasons that J. be part of what is said. You can help J. get the most out of classroom discussion either by repeating what is said into the FM microphone or by passing the microphone around so that each of the children can speak directly into it. I understand that this will require more effort on your part, but it will be very helpful to J. and may even be helpful to other children who have missed what was said by children who speak in a soft voice.

To be certain that J. gets correct assignments, it would be helpful if assignments were written down rather than given verbally. This will also be helpful to other children in the class who may have learning or attention difficulties.

There may be times when J. does not understand what you are saying. Try to repeat it. If it is still not understood, try and rephrase it. Sometimes, saying it in other words will help. Do not shout or overarticulate. Shouting and exaggerating your mouth movements only make it more difficult to lipread and to hear.

Talking about Hearing Loss

No child likes to feel different and most hearing-impaired children don't want to attract attention to their hearing aids or FM systems. However, it is not possible to hide a hearing loss. You can help J. accept his hearing loss and at the same time help the other children in the classroom understand that some children are different but that each of us is valuable. We have found that this is best handled in a very direct way. We suggest that you lead a discussion about how we are all different: some of us are tall, some are short, some wear eyeglasses and some wear hearing aids. Children are usually helpful when they are directed to be so. They can be asked to face J. when speaking and to try not to shout but simply to repeat something if it was not understood. They can be asked to take turns to be certain that J. receives assignments and knows what page is being referred to. If possible, it might help to have the children listen to the hearing aid or FM so they can hear what it sounds like. We can provide you with listening tubes to help with this. There are a number of good children's books dealing with this topic that we can lend to you.

Thank you for helping. If we can be of help in any way, please do not hesitate to call us. We will be happy to come to the school and provide you with assistance, if needed.

Sincerely,

Audiologist

APPENDIX 12

What To Look for in a School Visit

Use of Amplification

1. Is the child using personal amplification appropriately?
2. Does the child know how to use classroom amplification appropriately?
3. Does the teacher know how to use classroom amplification appropriately? When to turn it on and off?

Classroom Noise

1. Is the classroom in a quiet area of the school?
   Does it face a highly trafficked street?
   Is in next to the gym? the bathrooms? the music room?
2. Do chairs and table have rubber feet to reduce noise?
3. Is there carpeting, at least in the block or shop corner?
4. Is the classroom an "open" classroom with more than one class in the room?

Child's Seating Placement

1. Is the child seated in the best place for all activities?
2. Can the child's seat be changed during the day if the teacher moves for different activities?
3. Is the child facing away from lighting glare?

Child's Communication and Socialization Skills

1. Does the child understand and follow the teacher's conversation?
2. Does the teacher understand the child?

3. Does the child understand other children?
4. Do other children understand the child?
5. Does the child participate in classroom discussion?
6. Does the child play with other children? Does she or he have friends?
7. Do other children seek out the hearing-impaired child during play?
8. How does the child make his or her wants known?
9. Does the child appear comfortable in the room?
10. How does the child communicate?
    By listening? speechreading? cued speech? sign? combination?
11. Do the teacher and other students understand how the child communicates best?

The Teacher

1. Does the teacher face the child when he or she speaks?
   Does the teacher's articulation permit easy speechreading?
2. Does the teacher check that the hearing-impaired child understands?
3. How does the teacher ensure that the child is following classroom conversation?
   Does the teacher repeat classroom conversation into the FM mic or pass the mic around?
4. Does the teacher alert the child to changes in topic, etc.
5. Are assignments written down?
6. Does the teacher feel comfortable with a hearing-impaired child in the room?
7. Does the teacher have realistic expectations? Are they too high or too low?

Additional Assistance

1. Would the child benefit from having a "buddy" to help in knowing the topic, etc?
2. Does the child need additional tutoring?
3. Does the child need preteaching?
4. Does the child need an interpreter (oral, cued-speech, sign)?
5. Would the child benefit from a notetaker?
6. Does the child need a classroom aide?
7. Is this the appropriate class placement?

Other School Personnel

1. Do other school personnel know how to communicate with the hearing-impaired child?
2. Do special-subject teachers know how to use the FM system?
3. Who is assigned to monitor and check the FM system?
   Is there a backup person?

APPENDIX 13

Family Request List

I would like more information about

_____ My child's hearing loss

      _____ What is my child's hearing loss?

      _____ What caused the hearing loss?

      _____ Will it change?

_____ How does a hearing aid work?

      _____ How can I be sure that these hearing aids are right for my child?

      _____ How much should hearing aids be worn?

      _____ Can a hearing aid hurt?

      _____ How much will hearing aids help?

      _____ How will my child learn to listen with hearing aids?

_____ How will my child learn to speak?

      _____ How can I communicate with my child?

      _____ How long will it take for therapy to start helping?

_____ Other _____

I would like more information about

_____ Causes of hearing loss

_____ Hearing aids and FM systems

_____ Hearing test methods

_____ Different communication systems for hearing-impaired children

      _____ American Sign Language

      _____ Signing Exact English

_____ Cued speech

_____ Total communication

_____ Oral education

_____ Auditory–verbal therapy

_____ Different educational programs for hearing-impaired children

_____ Mainstreaming

_____ Inclusion

_____ Resource room

_____ Special class in regular school

_____ School for the deaf

I would like to have

_____ the names and phones number of other families with hearing-impaired children

_____ Another family with a hearing-impaired child call me

_____ Information about parent meetings for families with hearing-impaired children

_____ Lists of reading materials

_____ Names of organizations for hearing-impaired children and their families

_____ Other _____

APPENDIX 14

Genetic Evaluation and Counseling for the Hearing Impaired

The Purpose of a Genetic Evaluation

An individual or family may wish to see a geneticist for a variety of reasons. In the case of hearing loss, common questions are how genetic factors could cause hearing loss, whether there are any associated medical complications, whether the hearing loss might progress, and what the chances are that another family member might be born with or develop hearing loss. In order to give the most accurate answers to these questions, a genetic evaluation is done to try to determine the cause of the hearing loss.

Hearing loss may be caused by things that are not genetic, such as infection, but in about 50% of cases of severe to profound deafness, the cause is genetic. There are many different types of genetic conditions. They may be "syndromic", involving other medical or physical findings in addition to the hearing loss, or "non-syndromic", meaning that there are no other significant features besides the hearing loss. There are several ways in which hearing loss can be inherited: autosomal dominant, autosomal recessive, X-linked (dominant or recessive), multifactorial, or chromosomal. Genetic hearing loss may be present at birth ("congenital") or it may start later in life. It may be stable or progressive; it may be conductive, sensorineural, or mixed.

What Happens in a Genetic Evaluation

Physical Examination

The genetic evaluation is usually done by a team made up of a geneticist, a physician specially trained to recognize signs of genetic conditions, and a counselor who either has a Masters degree or Ph.D. in genetics. The medical history (including records from the audiologist and Ear-Nose-and-Throat doctor) and family history are reviewed and a specialized physical examination is performed. The medical history may identify a medical cause of hearing loss such as a serious illness, an injury, or an infection the mother had in pregnancy, or it may point out an important symptom of a genetic condition, such as kidney infections or difficulty seeing in the dark. A careful physical examination is done to look for subtle characteristics that can be related to specific genetic conditions. These characteristics by themselves may not be abnormalities, and they may appear to be unrelated to hearing loss. For example, small pits in front of the ears could indicate branchio-oto-renal syndrome, which also involves kidney problems; a white forelock could be part of Waardenburg syndrome; nightblindness or tunnel vision could indicate Usher syndrome, or severe nearsightedness could be a sign of Stickler syndrome.

Family History

The counselor goes over the family history and draws a "family tree", usually covering about three generations. For example, in the case of a child with hearing loss, the family history information would cover the child's brothers and sisters, parents and grandparents, and aunts, uncles, and cousins. Any relative with hearing loss is noted, along with any other physical or learning problems they may have had. In addition, there are a number of specific conditions that should be asked about in any relative, whether or not they have hearing loss. This is because syndromes include one or more additional findings in addition to the hearing loss. A person with a syndrome does not necessarily have all of the findings. Thus, the counselor will ask about such things as kidney problems, ear pits, white forelocks, nightblindness, nearsightedness, and so on.

Medical Testing

Typically, both parents and any brothers and sisters are asked to have audiological testing, and medical reports or tests may be needed from other family members as well. In addition, the geneticist may recommend specific medical tests such as ultrasound of the kidneys, an X-ray, or a blood or urine test. An examination by an ophthalmologist is often recommended (if it has not been done already), and an ERG (electroretinogram) may be done to screen for Usher syndrome, which also involves progressive visual problems due to retinitis pigmentosa. An EKG (electrocardiogram) may be done to look for a specific abnormality in the heartbeat that is seen in the Jervell and Lange-Nielsen syndrome. This would be done especially if there is any history of fainting. A CAT scan, which is a type of X-ray, may be recommended in order to look at the structure of the middle ear, cochlea, and vestibular system. An ABR (auditory brainstem response; sometimes called a BER, or brainstem evoked response) can be done to detect a hearing loss in a baby or a person who cannot perform a regular behavioral audiological evaluation. The ABR can also see if a sensorineural hearing problem lies in the cochlea, the auditory nerve, or in the part of the brain that first receives the sound information. Vestibular testing can tell if the vestibular system in the inner ear which contributes to the sense of balance has been affected as well. In some genetic forms of hearing loss, the vestibular system may not have developed, and meningitis can also damage the vestibular system. In a very young child, tests for viral infections may show that the child had a congenital infection (that is, an infection before birth) such as CMV (cytomegalovirus) or rubella which could have caused the hearing loss. Blood and urine tests that look at kidney function are also important because of the genetic conditions that involve both the ears and kidneys. A blood test for thyroid function may be done to screen for Pendred syndrome, which includes goiter.

Genetic Testing

Chromosome tests may be done in some cases when a person has other physical or developmental problems. Chromosomes are the tiny pieces of DNA in each cell of the body that carry the genes. The chromosomes can be examined under the microscope to see if a chromosome or part of a chromosome is missing or duplicated. However, in order for an abnormality to be seen under the microscope, it must be fairly large and involve many genes. At this time, geneticists cannot see individual genes, such as the gene for Waardenburg syndrome, so this test cannot be used to diagnose a hearing loss caused by a single gene.

The Results of the Evaluation

If It's Genetic

When the whole evaluation process has been completed, the results are explained to the family. If the hearing loss is genetic, the way it is inherited will be discussed. If a syndrome is identified, the geneticist describes the medical or physical features, and if there are any, concerns for future medical problems and how they can be managed. In some cases, there are support groups for individuals or families with the syndrome.

If It's Still Unknown

Unfortunately, the cause of the hearing loss may still be unknown even after an extensive medical genetic evaluation. This is particularly true when there is only one person in the family with hearing loss, and neither they nor anyone else in the family have any of the signs of a syndrome. In this case, the hearing loss might have been caused by something which is not genetic, but it also could be genetic. The most common genetic cause would be autosomal recessive inheritance, in which the person with the hearing loss has two genes for hearing loss. Each of the parents would have only one gene for hearing loss, which would not affect their hearing. They would have inherited that gene from one of their parents, and so on back through generations; only when both parents have the gene, and both pass it on to a child, would the hearing loss show up. There would be a 25% chance with each pregnancy that they could have a child with hearing loss. A person with autosomal recessive hearing loss would have a very small chance of having a child with hearing loss, unless they married someone with exactly the same genes for hearing loss or with a dominant form of hearing loss.

It would also be possible that a person with hearing loss could have a dominant gene that is new to him or her and which arose through the process of mutation. No one else in the family, including the parents, would have the gene, but the person with the new hearing loss gene would have a 50% chance of passing it on to a child. Finally, if the person with the hearing loss is a male, it is possible that the hearing loss is X-linked. The mother could "carry" the gene, or it could have appeared for the first time in the boy with hearing loss.

What Is the Chance It Will Occur Again?

Even when the cause of the hearing loss remains unknown, the family can be given estimates of the chance it will recur in another relative. These estimated risks are based on studies of many families with similar family histories. For example, if the family is a hearing couple who has had one child who is profoundly deaf, the chance that the next child would be deaf is about 10% [F.R. Bieber & W.E. Nance. 1978. L.G. Jackson, R.N. Schimke, (Eds) Clinical Genetics: A source book for Physicians. NY; Wiley.] If both parents are deaf, and the cause of their deafness is unknown, the chance that their first child would be deaf would also be about 10%.

This brings up some very important points about genetic counseling. Genetics professionals in the United States support the idea of "non-directive" counseling, which means that genetic counseling is meant to be informative and supportive. It is not meant to tell people what to do or whether or not to have children. These principles have been adopted by the major professional societies for genetics professionals.

Different Perspectives

Particularly in the case of hearing loss, people may have quite different attitudes about deafness in their family. For example, some hearing parents might be concerned about having another child who is deaf, while others may feel that the hearing loss would not pose a problem, but would want to know if any other medical problems might be involved. Similarly, deaf parents may feel comfortable about their own abilities, but would prefer not to have a deaf child, whereas other deaf parents may be more concerned about the challenges of raising a hearing child.

Date Originally Created: Fall of 1990.

The information presented here first appeared in publications of the Boys Town National Research Register for Hereditary Hearing Loss, the National Institute on Deafness and Other Communication Disorders (NIDCD), Hereditary Hearing Impairment Resource Registry (HHIRR), or the Boys Town Research Registry for Hereditary Hearing Loss.

WWW URL: http://www.boystown.org/deafgene.registry/

Index

Page numbers in *italics* indicate figures. Page numbers followed by "t" indicate tables.